BodyMindMovement

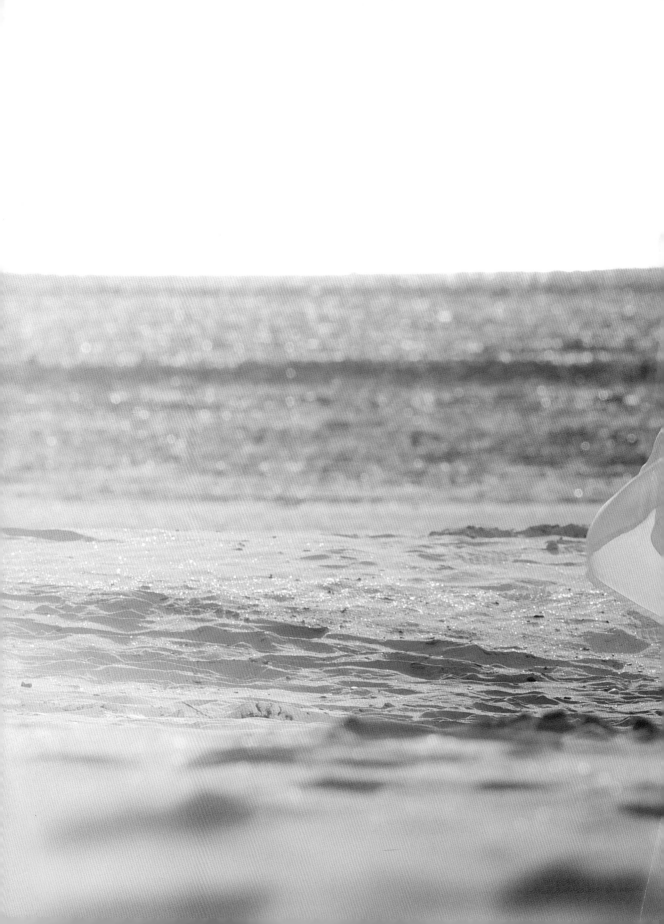

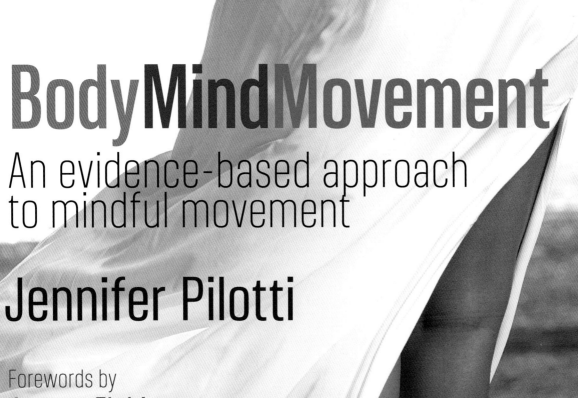

BodyMindMovement

An evidence-based approach to mindful movement

Jennifer Pilotti

Forewords by
Joanne Elphinston
Christine Ruffolo
Kathryn Bruni-Young

HANDSPRING
PUBLISHING
Edinburgh

HANDSPRING PUBLISHING LIMITED
The Old Manse, Fountainhall,
Pencaitland, East Lothian
EH34 5EY, United Kingdom
Tel: +44 1875 341 859
Website: www.handspringpublishing.com

First published 2020 in the United Kingdom by Handspring Publishing

ISBN 978-1-912085-89-7
ISBN (Kindle eBook) 978-1-912085-90-3

British Library Cataloguing in Publication Data
A catalogue record for this book is available from the British Library

Library of Congress Cataloguing in Publication Data
A catalog record for this book is available from the Library of Congress

Notice
Neither the Publisher nor the Authors assume any responsibility for any loss or injury and/or damage to persons or property arising out of or relating to any use of the material contained in this book. It is the responsibility of the treating practitioner, relying on independent expertise and knowledge of the patient, to determine the best treatment and method of application for the patient.

All reasonable efforts have been made to obtain copyright clearance for illustrations in the book for which the authors or publishers do not own the rights. If you believe that one of your illustrations has been used without such clearance please contact the publishers and we will ensure that appropriate credit is given in the next reprint.

Commissioning Editor Sarena Wolfaard
Copy Editor Kathryn Mason Pak
Project Manager Morven Dean
Designer Bruce Hogarth
Photography Michelle Robertson
Indexer Aptara, India
Typesetter DiTech Process Solutions
Printer Finidr, Czech Republic

The
Publisher's
policy is to use
paper manufactured
from sustainable forests

CONTENTS

FOREWORD *by Joanne Elphinston*

The experience of ourselves as a lived body is most directly encountered through our movement. With *Body Mind Movement*, Jennifer Pilotti issues a thoughtful invitation to movement practitioners to join her in a truly holistic and highly accessible exploration of the science and practice of movement teaching.

This is a book about connection at a deeply personal level. It is about the awareness that reveals unsuspected alternatives in our experience of ourselves, an unfolding process that connects and clarifies our present state with acute clarity and, in doing so, challenges our assumptions about our futures as inhabitants and users of our own bodies.

To become aware involves a complex interplay of systems, but it begins with startling simplicity, in a state of quiet contemplation. As Jennifer herself says, "Movement creates more movement, even if the movement is subtle at first." Subtlety is a rare and often undervalued quality. To achieve it requires an understanding of a great many factors if the practitioner is to truly meet the needs of each individual they encounter. Jennifer explains the relationships between these factors with elegance, guiding the reader through potentially complex physiology and neurology with a gentle hand.

Body Mind Movement offers invaluable insights into the relationship between pain perception, beliefs and movement behavior, mining rich resources of neuroscience. With her easy, conversational style, Jennifer explains this potentially complex material in a way that increases confidence in the reader, just as she recommends they do with their own clients. For those working with clients with pain or an injury history, her suggestions regarding mindset, language, and the creation of a sense of safe achievability accurately reflect contemporary rehabilitation research in an accessible, pragmatic way. What emerges is the gift of possibility, where restrictive conventional practices are challenged and a more flexible, responsive and personal conception of movement training and recovery shimmers into view.

Jennifer's approach takes the learner beyond "Where am I?" to "What is it like to be here right now?" With less effort expended on worrying whether relative body positions are correct, the learner starts to forge a new relationship with themselves, based on their felt experience. This confers greater self-responsibility for investigating other possibilities, but also the liberty to explore those new choices with curiosity rather than criticism. For many people, this is a surprising experience. When invited to notice the feel, shape, and dimensions of their own strategies, they become aware of themselves, and, in so doing, come to understand and take ownership of their body's opportunities. Thus, variability becomes possible, and a new landscape of options appears.

Drawing from her own extensive experience, Jennifer provides both case studies to illustrate the practical application of the principles she presents and easy self-explorations to encourage the reader to step past the words on the page and into their own body. In a field which is often attracted towards increasing complexity to solve its problems, Jennifer's quietly focused investigations, supported amply by their anatomical and biomechanical basis, are uncomplicated and unpretentious. This gives the nervous system space and time to notice itself, make new connections and challenge previous beliefs, perceptions and behaviors.

So many movement professionals are taught from the "outside in." They may speak the language of body awareness, but their concern is largely *where* the body is rather than *how* the body is. Focus is not the same thing as awareness, leading to concentration being mistaken for mindfulness. Jennifer's simple tasks allow a client to encounter themselves in a safe and non-judgmental way, learning about the relationship between their body structure and its movement, truly from the inside out,

Foreword

as they learn to connect with their own proprioceptive and interoceptive feedback. It is a skill for living, a path back to movement spontaneity, and an antidote to the sense of helplessness that so many people experience when suffering from pain or the aftermath of an accident or injury.

Jennifer's translation of the science of movement into this quiet, powerful and – above all – kind book, will support the work of any holistically minded movement professional as they inspire their own clients to reclaim their future physicality.

Joanne Elphinston
Author of *The Power and the Grace*
Creator of the JEMS® rehabilitation and
performance approach

Cardiff, UK
April, 2020

FOREWORD *by Christine Ruffolo*

"Death to Exercise, Long Live Movement!" The chants get louder and louder. Exercise, this mindless, made-up thing to counter our sedentary and convenient lifestyles, is and always has been a distraction from ourselves. It stood and still stands an isolated moment of personal punishment or penance, a way of being "good" so we can make up for our "bad." But what if we could look at our patterns of behavior without judgment? What if instead of labeling something as right or wrong, we saw it as it is, as it *really* is? How much more informed might we be, and what might we be able to do with that information?

Jenn Pilotti aims to prepare you to answer this question through these pages. With science and studies as her sword, she hands it to you as if it were a shield, cutting out all of the extraneous noise and non-applicable banter that leaves the reader uncertain and unmoved. What is left is *you*, realizing that you just might already have all the things you need. We just need a little help recognizing what to pay attention to.

The *movement* is really about your understanding of yourself and how you work. There are subtle signals that your body tries to tell you every day, all the time. Following what Jenn points out is the first step to knowing how to listen, feel, adjust, and appreciate. *You are a marvel.* Imagine how you might carry and interact with yourself if you found yourself the most interesting thing in the world?

As with any idea that contradicts mainstream views and upsets the status quo, presentation determines whether it will be deemed acceptable or not. How does it fit with what people already hold to be true? Each chapter starts with a Case Study that sets up a narrative about mental components being affective to a person's physical being. A story (footnoted by studies) sets the scene. The first half outlines the relationship between noticing and feeling: what to look for, how the brain and body utilize and can get stuck in feedback loops, and what one can do to break them from detrimental patterns. Each align with "learn by doing" activities that teach you concepts via *sensation*. Brilliantly bridged by balance, the second half of the book looks at troubleshooting common problem areas, guiding you through *applying the principles* outlined in the first half. "Things to Consider and Observe," the excellent inquisitive ending for each section, leaves you wondering and wanting to come up with examinations of your own.

Therein lies *Mindful Movement's* greatest success - to start looking with fascination at all the things you might have missed. When care and attention is given to normal things, they quickly become extraordinary. The same holds true for people. The separation between teacher and student comes in the form of who asks and answers questions. In the case of Jenn Pilotti, she can seamlessly toggle between both.

Christine Ruffolo, BS Kinesiology, MA Teaching
Physical education teacher, Woodburn High School
Movement therapist

Salem, Oregon
April, 2020

FOREWORD *by Kathryn Bruni-Young*

I believe if every teacher and trainer learned this material as part of their education, we would not only move differently but treat our students differently. *Body Mind Movement* will teach you how to get in touch with the layers of movement that we usually brush over as well as how sensing and feeling can change the way we move.

Jennifer Pilotti has effectively articulated some of the most interesting aspects of human movement. Her work combines moving with feeling and sensing, which are oftentimes lost in mainstream exercise culture. It's teachers like Jenn who are moving this industry to a more inquiry-based approach, which takes into account not only muscles and joints but the nervous system, feelings, pain, emotions, and every part of the human experience. The books of this decade are going to change the way teachers and trainers work with their students, and this one helps us understand that there is more to exercise than the exercises.

In addition to providing the necessary nuance on misunderstood topics like posture and sitting, *Body Mind Movement* creates a new framework for how to understand and assess the body. It will teach you not only the value of structured varied movement but how to explore your options. Jenn brings evidence to life with creative exercises and ways of working and being in the body. From breath to personal safety, motor learning, and basic exercises like squatting, we learn that being in the body is vital to healthy movement. Jenn will teach you how to connect with your body in a down-to-earth way. The exercises she presents are perfectly balanced in accessibility, research, and personal exploration.

In a community that is steeped in specific alignment rules and dogmatic thinking about movement, these ideas are even more important. Jenn's work presents the information and empowers the reader to be in touch with their experience without emphasizing a right or wrong way to move. I'm certain this book will be included in many movement training classrooms – it can be applied to asana, personal training, gym class, and beyond.

Kathryn Bruni-Young
International yoga and movement teacher

Ontario, Canada
April, 2020

ABOUT THE AUTHOR

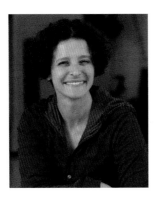

Jennifer Pilotti, MS, has been teaching movement to people of all ages and abilities for over 17 years. She is passionate about helping people feel comfortable, strong, mobile, and capable in their bodies using concepts rooted in proprioception, mindset, the science of learning, and motor control.

She has a special interest in the effect of movement on mental health: specifically on anxiety, chronic pain, and trauma.

She implements techniques from a variety of disciplines, including yoga, strength and conditioning, Feldenkrais, dance, gymnastics, and Natural Movement. She teaches workshops and online courses, and regularly writes about the concepts that comprise the foundations of awareness, mobility, and strength.

Jenn owns a personal training studio, where she works with people aged 12–95, creating individualized interventions that are designed to inspire curiosity and enhance well-being. To learn more about Jenn's in-person workshops and retreats, please visit www.jennpilotti.com.

I began writing about movement to help me make sense of what I experienced, both as a movement professional and as a movement practitioner. In the days before weekend trainings were abundant and YouTube held all of the answers about different exercise options, I found myself reading, experimenting, and conflicted about the best way to move.

This inner conflict slowly gave way to a relaxed state of curiosity as I realized helping people feel more at home in their bodies didn't have to be predicated on a specific set of postural rules or regimented biomechanics. I realized that when people were given space to explore and they didn't feel overly concerned about performing a movement "right," they became more curious and playful in their approach to movement and their bodies. This curiosity led to less fear around injury and sensation.

I began to learn from my clients by watching as they self-organized in ways that worked for them. I paid attention to their words and actions, learning from their stories and experiences. I slowly began to let go of the idea that a perfect, prescriptive set of exercises existed that would suddenly make everyone feel embodied, capable, and strong. I began to realize that understanding basic tenets of how the experience of movement affects the emotional self made me a better teacher and a more empathetic and compassionate practitioner.

As I stumbled down the rabbit hole of movement sciences, researching and learning about a wide variety of topics under the mind/body umbrella, I came to realize that posture, breathing, and freedom of movement are by-products of feeling safe and appropriately challenged. Moving in a coordinated way involves slowing down, feeling, and listening.

The more I explored these ideas in the studio, the more I felt compelled to share what I was learning by writing. The writing process clarified concepts and forced me to examine the gaps in my knowledge and understanding, especially when the evidence was contrary to my beliefs. And so I studied more and became more comfortable with the fact that movement is a multi-sensory experience, that balance, proprioception, and mindset all factor in to how we engage with the world. I learned that understanding the basic walking pattern was a way to identify holes in body schema and kinesthetic awareness, and that strength and breathing could both affect a change in tension and the feeling of stability.

Movement is an integration of senses, senses that can be developed with practice, focused attention, and play. Moving well isn't about moving right; rather, it's about exploring coordination, tapping into it subtly, and integrating the entire physical system into an experience that makes us feel whole. The following pages are the foundation of my work helping people feel – and tap into – the lost sense of embodiment through the cultivation of awareness.

Jennifer Pilotti
April, 2020

ACKNOWLEDGMENTS

Though writing is a solitary pursuit, it takes the support of many for the process to come to life. Below are some of the people who helped me along the way.

Thank you to Annie, Pat, and Paula for encouraging me to turn my ideas into a book. It took a while, but, eventually, I listened.

Thank you, Bobbie, for your optimism, support, and expertise with the English language. I am eternally grateful for your feedback and what I learned.

Thank you, Dainen, for giving me the space to write, research, and edit. At times it was all encompassing, and you were incredibly patient.

To all of the students and clients I have had the privilege to work with over the last 18 years, thank you. I wrote that movement is experiential; so, too, is teaching, and there were times I was learning by doing. Witnessing the commitment, consistency, and willingness to try gave me the courage to keep pursuing an alternative path.

And, of course, to everyone reading this book, thank you for being curious, for examining the effect that movement can have on not just the body, but the whole person.

INTRODUCTION

When I graduated from college in 2002, equipped with an exercise physiology degree, a nationally recognized certification, two years working in labs, hospitals, and gyms, and a full-time job offer as a personal trainer, I felt confident I could change lives by making people stronger, fitter, and more flexible. I quickly realized I was much less prepared than I anticipated to work with people across a wide spectrum of ages and with varying degrees of body awareness. In those early years, I often felt like an imposter posing as a fitness and movement professional because, really, I had no idea what I was actually doing.

And so I went searching, taking to the Internet to answer all of my questions about the things I saw, attempting to understand what they meant and how to change them. I began acquainting myself with other disciplines, trying to understand why certain techniques worked, why others worked less often, and what made someone great at teaching movement.

I became frustrated by what I felt was a lack of transparency regarding the underlying principles of teaching movement, strength, and mobility. I also began to realize that in an attempt to make information more accessible, movement characteristics were itemized and people were placed into categories based on how they performed specific movements or held specific postures. This, I began to see, ignored the whole person. A person's movement patterns are more than just a tight this and a weak that. Movement patterns represent past experiences, beliefs, and emotional states. They aren't simply a biomechanics representation of ability.

As I dove further into psychology and pain science, I began to realize that while the fundamental concepts behind teaching movement effectively aren't complicated, people are complicated. Listening to people's stories and watching spontaneous movement was more powerful than an itemized assessment for gathering information about how a person interpreted movement.

I continued to study, determined to understand what allowed people to move freely in a coordinated, integrated way. I went to graduate school and attended workshops, exposing myself to several systems and modalities. I spent countless hours reading research papers and textbooks on different, but related topics. What I finally came to understand was this: helping people feel more of their body led to more integrated movement. Kinesthetic awareness, proprioception, and understanding and applying the principles of learning in a movement setting elicited long-term changes in movement habits, strength, and mobility. Nothing trumps consistency if the goal is to become more flexible and strong in the long term, but consistency performed with an element of mindfulness makes people curious. This curiosity changes a person's relationship to movement by blending the physical act of movement with the realization that how you think about movement changes how it is expressed, ultimately leading to a more embodied existence.

The first four chapters outline the foundations of mindful movement, drawing on concepts from psychology, motor control, neuroscience, and biomechanics. The last five chapters apply the concepts through an exploration of different aspects of the body and how these different parts connect. Since movement is experiential, there are exercises throughout each chapter designed to implement putting the science into practice.

Understanding concepts gives you, the teacher, an opportunity to apply the concepts in a way that resonates with you and is appropriate for the person in front of you. One of the things that became clear to me as I navigated the murky waters of movement science is that there is no perfect system, but there are excellent teachers: people with the ability to communicate, teach, and implement the foundations of movement science in a seamless way that creates connection. Ultimately, this newly established connection between the mind and body leads to a change in a person's ability to coordinate and understand movement.

When a person becomes more coordinated and comfortable in the body they inhabit, the ability to move in a freer way emerges. The more someone moves in a variety of ways, the stronger and more flexible the person becomes. Movement creates more movement, and this, I think, is the reason movement matters, the reason movement teachers exist, and the reason I spent more than a decade trying to understand why things worked. The opposite of movement is stillness, but even during stillness, the breath creates movement, so during life, we are never really completely still. Life, like movement, is meant to be experienced; by gaining confidence in your skills as a teacher and learning how to implement basic concepts so you can work with almost anyone creates a forward momentum that impacts far more than someone's physical state.

The beauty of taking the time to study the basic principles outlined in the following chapters is that it demystifies the process of effective movement teaching, making it more accessible in a variety of settings. Mindful movement can be taught in any setting involving physical movement. Join me in exploring how.

How to access the online videos

Short tutorials that complement chapters 4-9 of this book are available online for free. For students who are interested in further understanding and practical application of the material, please visit:

https://awareness-mobility-strength.teachable.com/p/mindful-movement or go via the QR link below using the password MMBOOK2020 at checkout.

The QR code can be scanned with a smart phone using an app, and many free apps are available to download. If you are using an iPad or iPhone running the latest software (iOS 11 or higher) then no additional app is required. Simply open your camera and point it at the code (no need to take a picture). A notification should pop down from the top and then tap that and you will be taken to the video.

Case study

Jean came in to see me because she had persistent back pain. She owns a shop that requires her to stand and move around throughout the day.

I observed Jean as we spoke, and I noticed she had a tendency to lean back, arching her chest forward. We did a few things and I noticed this was her tendency every time she stood still. She had developed a habit of leaning back in order to "stand up straight."

I had her shift her weight forward so her torso came forward over her hips. This immediately lessened the arch in her back. Then I had her move the ribs toward the floor by exhaling, bringing her chest down and centering her weight over her feet. Her persistent back pain in the "new" position was suddenly gone.

I told her that I wanted her to practice observing her standing position when she was at work or waiting in line. If she noticed her back was achy, I told her to shift her torso position and see if she could find a place that was more comfortable, or use her exhale to shift her rib position. "What you perceive as standing up straight is actually leaning back," I explained to her.

This was enlightening for Jean, and the next time she came in, she reported less back discomfort during standing. "Whenever I would notice it, I would shift my position, and most of the time, it worked." As Jean's awareness about how she held herself in her daily life continued to grow, she began to feel more ease. Her discomfort continued to decrease, and, while she needed to gain strength and mobility to help her feel more stable as she moved through her day, altering her position and checking in with herself occasionally created an opportunity for connecting with her body. Her habitual standing pressure wasn't wrong or harmful; however, she had become sensitized to it, which means it was causing discomfort. Her perception of where she was in space was also altered. Her sense of straight was actually leaning back. Giving her options for her position also gave her an opportunity to enhance her body schema.

When things like stiffness or pain are viewed as permanent situations, then that is what they will become. If you ask your clients and students to become active observers of their discomfort through inquiry, you are empowering them by giving them control over their bodies and their positions. Asking, "What happens if you change the way you're moving or holding yourself?" is very different than telling someone their posture is potentially injurious.

How do your clients view the physical sensations they experience on a regular basis? When clients have an ache or pain that persists regularly, do they tell you, "I can't go down stairs because it bothers my knees"? Or maybe they tell you, "My back is bad so there are certain exercises I can't do."

The acceptance of certain physical conditions and the assumption that a person's current physical state is their forever state is an example of a fixed mindset. The potential trouble with a fixed mindset is it reduces intrinsic motivation. Intrinsic motivation is related to motivation, curiosity, and the desire to learn throughout the lifespan (Ng 2018). If there is reduced curiosity about physical skills and a decrease in confidence navigating the physical world, an individual's movement options begin to decrease. Things like difficulty balancing or not feeling strong can lead to anxiety (Gordon et al. 2017; Shefer et al. 2014), resulting in the cessation of certain activities because of a reduced sense of trust in the body's physical capabilities.

How you talk with your clients and students can have a direct impact on their mindset. How can you choose words or cues that shift their thinking? What if instead of emphasizing muscle groups or contraction and relaxation,

continued

Chapter 1

you incorporated cues and movements that demonstrated that body parts and muscles don't function in an isolated way? What if instead of suggesting pain was a permanent state and indicative of a biomechanical issue, you asked students to be curious about their sensations and explore different positions or different ways of performing a movement, observing how changing the load in the tissues could potentially alter their experience? Persistent joint and nerve pain should, of course, receive medical attention, but so much of what people perceive as pain is feedback from the neuromuscular system saying, "Hey, can you consider shifting the weight elsewhere so the load is dispersed across a different area?" I invite you to consider that the way your clients and students experience balance, coordination, and breathing, and the way they use their body could be changed because they are capable of learning; one of your jobs as a movement teacher is to ask the right questions and offer opportunities for learning.

Researcher and psychology professor Carol Dweck writes in her book, *Mindset: The New Psychology of Success*, "In fact, every word and action can send a message. It tells children – or students, or athletes – how to think about themselves. It can be a fixed-mindset message that says: You have permanent traits and I'm judging them. Or it can be a growth-mindset message that says:

You are a developing person and I am committed to your development" (Dweck 2006: 173). She has spent her career studying mindset, specifically how our beliefs influence our motivation. Understanding growth versus fixed mindsets can help you understand how students view their world and their physical abilities. How you speak about movement and their movement will influence their beliefs about their ability to improve body awareness, mobility, and strength.

People begin a movement program because they want to change something, or explore a different way of using their bodies. This indicates they arrive primed with a desire to change. However, they don't always have a clear picture of their body and how it moves in space. They don't view body awareness as a skill to be learned and instead are simply seeking a physical change in weight, strength, or function. Showing people through the right inputs that they are capable of altering their behaviors/actions/physical state reinforces the fact that they have the capacity to learn and change with practice and hard work, instilling a growth mindset around the physical self. This makes it easier to recover from setbacks such as injury; it also makes movement interesting and (it is hoped) incites a desire to continue to explore movement throughout the lifespan.

A (brief) overview of how the brain and movement are interrelated

Let's pretend you decide you want to pick up a grocery bag. Your brain makes this decision before your body begins to carry out the physical act of reaching for the bag (Mosconi et al. 2015). Once the decision has been made, deep inside the recesses of your brain, your brain communicates with your body via the nervous system to find out what options are available for picking up the bag. If you always pick up the bag with your right hand, your brain takes the information from the afferent (sensing) nervous system and spits out information via the motor nervous system about how to execute the task. The limbs and the muscles will carry out the act of picking up the bag. All of this happens so fast it's unconscious and feels automatic.

And it is. If you had to think about every single movement you were making, you would be mentally exhausted and you would get a lot less done.

The central nervous system is comprised of the brain and the spinal cord. It's divided into two branches: the sensory (afferent) nervous system and the motor (efferent) nervous system. We will discuss this in more detail in Chapter 2, but, for now, you just need to know that, with regard to the nervous system, the afferent branch is the information-gathering part and the efferent branch is the reacting part. There are a lot of things that affect the information you gather and the brain's interpretation of the information.

Occasionally, the brain will receive information that certain movements, or that a specific body part, hurts. Let's pretend your right arm is bothering you and you aren't sure why. And let's pretend for the purposes of this example the pain is vague, a nagging irritation in the upper arm that's a bit diffuse. You can't quite figure out how to get it to go away, and, because of your background, you throw a lot of things at it like massage and corrective exercises. When you go to the doctor, they diagnose you with an overuse injury, which is a little perplexing, because you aren't sure how you are suddenly overusing the right arm. You begin to worry there is something more serious going on, even though the imaging comes back normal.

What if when the pain originally started, you began noticing how you used your right arm throughout the day and you noticed you always picked up things with your right arm, including the grocery bags? And what if when you noticed this, you began picking things up with your left arm occasionally to give your right arm a break? Maybe this slows you down a little bit, because you aren't used to picking things up with your left arm and your left arm can't lift as much because it's a little bit weaker than your right, but maybe this change to how you normally do things is enough to make your right arm feel better. Do you still feel there is something potentially wrong with your right arm?

I have worked with two clients in the last year who originally came to see me because of the scenario described above. Asking the right questions, focusing their attention on how they moved, asking them to use the left arm,

and giving them alternative movement options with the right arm caused a significant reduction in pain within a short amount of time. Creating an environment where it was okay to be curious about moving a different way also reframed their views of their shoulders, changing their narrative from "my right arm is bad/weak/injured" to "I can learn how to use my right arm differently and my left arm more."

What about posture?

Creating awareness about a person's physical habits is not the same thing as trying to create a certain position or posture. Motor control researchers define "posture" as stabilizing the body's center of mass and maintaining balance during internal and external perturbations (Dutt-Mazumder et al. 2018). A perturbation is a disturbance that alters position; posture is the place a person returns to after the disturbance. Even in quiet standing, there is something called postural sway, subtle movements the body makes to maintain its upright position. The neuromuscular system self-organizes, meaning it chooses how to stand based on previous experience, specifically what has worked well in the past. It also takes into account information it receives from your eyes, the vestibular system (the system that determines balance and orientation based on inner ear information), and the proprioceptive system (which gives the brain feedback about where the body is located in space through cells located in the muscles and joints) (Purves et al. 2001). We will explore all of these systems in greater detail in subsequent chapters.

Another way to view posture is as the transition between movements. It's the pause between being seated at a coffee shop and standing up to grab your bag. It's the moment before you roll over in bed, or before you swing your legs over to the side of the bed in preparation for getting up. It's the pause to glance out at the ocean before you resume walking.

Modern postural demands ask very little from us in terms of variability. Most people in developed countries work on hard surfaces, sit on soft surfaces, and sleep on soft surfaces. The density is consistent, which means our posture is consistent.

For some, the consistency in posture is heavily influenced by what others suggest we "should" be doing. At some point, good posture became synonymous with throwing the shoulders down and back and standing up "tall." These words sometimes backfire; interfering with the body's ability to self-organize can alter proprioception and kinesthetic awareness, aka the body's sense of where it is located in space and/or the internal image of what the body looks like.

This modern-day postural consistency is in contrast to how our ancestors likely navigated the environment. They stood and moved around on surfaces that weren't perfectly level and weren't always the same density. They sat on different surfaces, and they weren't able to choose which density they wanted for their pillow and mattresses. Their environment was varied, which means their posture was also varied and adaptable to a variety of situations.

Research is conflicting about whether posture corresponds to the development of pain (Murrie et al. 2003; Nourbakhsh & Arab 2002; Nakipoglu et al. 2008; Tavares et al. 2018; Wirth et al. 2018). But strong postural habits such as sitting the same way on the same chair, standing exactly the same way on similar surfaces, or driving in exactly the same position, can result in less movement variation. The body – and the brain – like variety, and by simply asking people to notice their tendencies, they will begin to create more of a connection to how they use their body throughout the day.

This doesn't mean that there aren't ways to maximize efficiency in specific positions. Depending on the goal of the task, different tactics can be used to increase the sensation of tension or increase the sensation of ease. For everyday tasks like standing and sitting, positions should not cause pain, should easily enable the individual to recover from an outside force or perturbation, and should be easy to move into and easy to move out of.

The brain has an internal image of the physical body. It's correlated to the amount of sensation (how much you can feel of the area) and how much time is spent moving each part. You may have seen a standard image that tends to represent this map: a cartoon-like figure called the homunculus man. The graphical illustration includes large lips, hands and feet, areas that are rich with sensory information.

The more you move and the more you use different body parts in an integrated way, the bigger each respective internal image becomes. These are your body maps and they represent your body schema, or your internal representation of what you look like (Holmes & Spence 2004). The more filled in your body maps are and the more accurate your body schema is, the more of yourself you will integrate unconsciously into everyday movement.

There are a number of things that affect body schema, including physical trauma, chronic pain, eating disorders, low self-esteem, cultural or social pressures, and disuse. Being aware of how an individual perceives their body schema can help the movement practitioner make a more informed decision in exercise selection.

Physical trauma occurs during things like surgery, falling, or previous injury. It can significantly impact how the brain incorporates the affected body part into daily activities. One study found older adults experienced a decrease in activities of daily living and an increase in pain following hip fracture and negative effects on mobility, body image, and mental health, indicating a change in body schema (Ehlers et al. 2018). Chronic pain, which is usually defined as pain persisting longer than three months, may be correlated with changes in body schema, altering how people use the painful limb in day-to-day activities (Ravat et al. 2019).

Eating disorders such as anorexia nervosa and bulimia often result in dysfunctional neural activity in the posterior parietal cortex, the area of the brain engaged with the representation of body schema. The internal representation of an individual with anorexia or bulimia reflects a mental image of body parts that are bigger than they actually are, affecting how they initiate and perform motor tasks (Purcell et al. 2018).

Self-esteem is how you feel about yourself; low self-esteem is characterized as a lack of confidence and feeling unlovable, awkward, and/or incompetent. A body-image disorder such as body dysmorphic disorder, a mental disorder characterized by obsession over a perceived flaw in appearance or in a physical defect, is associated with low self-esteem and is often considered an obsessive compulsive spectrum disorder, also resulting in an altered body schema (Bjornsson et al. 2010).

The emotional relationship with the physical body and self impacts an individual's perception of their movement capabilities. In one study, 100 healthy adult women were asked to predict what the smallest gap between sliding doors was that they could pass through. Women with low self-esteem and body image concerns were less accurate in their predictions than women with higher self-esteem (Irvine et al. 2019). How you feel about yourself and your emotional health affects your interpretation of how the physical self interacts with the world, and how your clients feel about themselves will influence how they move.

Cultural or social pressure to look a certain way or move a certain way can also influence body schema. Begin et al. (2019) found muscle dysmorphia, the excessive preoccupation with being muscular, was precipitated by social pressure to reach a muscular body in men with negative affect and narcissistic vulnerability. In a study that examined how women's perception of their body changed after breast cancer treatment in the country of Jordan, cancer survivors reported feeling like their bodies were broken and as though their future would be negatively impacted because of the cancer and its treatment (Alhusban 2019). Pressure to look a specific way, whether it's self-inflicted or socially inflicted, plays a role in body schema and self-perception, influencing how we generate movement. Movement patterns we deem socially acceptable become default patterns, habitual movements that slowly eliminate other movement options.

People who are inactive generally move in a less varied way. Research published in 2019 found a correlation between a sedentary lifestyle and nonspecific low back pain (low back pain that is chronic in nature with no specific cause) (Citko et al. 2018). Another study, published in 2018, found inactive individuals with neck pain had lower functional performance and lateral rotation of the shoulder, which correlated with neck pain intensity and catastrophizing (da Silva et al. 2018). Basically, the more varied your movements are on a regular basis, the more different parts of your body are incorporated into your body schema on a regular basis and the more confident you become in your physical capabilities.

Exercise
Interlocking the fingers

Interlock your fingers like you are holding your hands together. Look down and see which thumb is on top and how your fingers intertwine. Now, adjust the interlocking of the fingers so the opposite thumb is on top (Figure 1.1). How does that feel?

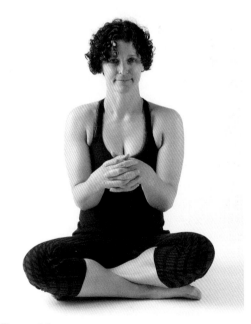

Figure 1.1

Chapter 1

Now, cross your arms across your chest so your hands touch the opposite shoulders. Which arm is on top?

Switch the arms so the other arm is on top (Figure 1.2). How does that feel?

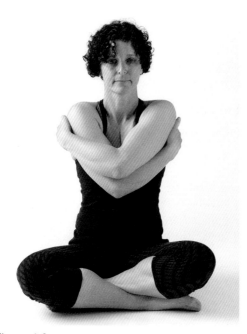

Figure 1.2

These two movements are easy ways to demonstrate potentially strong movement habits and/or altered body schemas. Clients sometimes tell me it feels like they are holding someone else's hand or they are crossing someone else's arms when I have them do drills like these. With practice, the "awkward" side becomes more familiar and they begin to use both sides of their bodies in a more varied way.

Everyone has a preferred way of doing specific tasks. As a result, it's not uncommon to use the dominant hand and arm one way and the non-dominant arm another way. Helping people become aware of their tendencies gives them the freedom to choose to move differently once in a while.

In extreme cases, one of the hands may feel a bit like a foreign object, as though it isn't part of the person. Imagine the image of the homunculus man. In this situation, the homunculus man lacks a clear outline of the foreign feeling hand. It's as though someone began drawing the outline of the hand and became distracted part way through, leaving the drawing to be filled in later.

This doesn't mean the non-dominant hand's body map can't be improved. It absolutely can. It does, however, mean the movement professional should choose their language carefully, not implying one side is "good" or "bad," and that the student will need to focus on identifying their normal movement habits and consciously pick alternative ways to move. This requires both effort and patience for both the teacher and the student.

When adjectives such as "good," "perfect," "better," "broken," "bad," and "uncooperative" are used to describe the behavior of the limbs and torso, or the body and its parts are viewed as incapable of change, the body becomes a physical aspect of the self that isn't viewed as strong, resilient, or intelligent. When a teacher suggests a movement is problematic in any way because it's bad for the back/knees/shoulders, or because it could potentially result in injury, that reinforces the idea that the body is a fragile structure. This doesn't mean throw safety to the wind – all exercises and skills should be progressed in a way that instills confidence and the necessary components of mobility and strength in order for the student to be successful. It does mean that the language chosen to describe the body and how it moves should be empowering, not fear-provoking.

Mindsets, just like the physical experience of the world, can be changed. If you are working with someone with strong ideas about the separation of the mind and the body, your job isn't to change their mind with words; rather, it's to show them with carefully chosen movements and inquiry that their bodies are strong and capable of moving differently. If you ask the right questions and choose tasks that both highlight movement habits and create opportunities for alternative paths of movement, the student will become interested in the physical aspect of self. This glimpses into the connection between the mind and the body and demonstrates the capacity they have to learn.

Case study

I began working with a woman who struggled with pain and anxiety. She had also lost a significant amount of weight and didn't feel connected to her new body – another way to put it is that she was disembodied.

She would frequently say derogatory things about her body, upset that it was letting her down. I would correct her language and help her rephrase, telling her that her shoulder wasn't stupid; it was part of her and just needed to learn how to do certain things differently. Her feet weren't bad, I told her; they supported her every day. They just needed to gain strength.

Over time, her dialog shifted. Whenever she would catch herself saying something that either created separation between the self and the body or was negative, she would rephrase. Slowly, she gained strength and confidence in her ability to move in ways that didn't reinforce painful outcomes.

It has been suggested that one of the reasons language developed was to explain perception, emotions, and action (Holmes & Spence 2004). When you perceive yourself as small, distances look farther away. When you are holding heavy bags, hills look steeper; but if you stepped on the scale and found out you lost three pounds, the hill will look less steep. The language used to describe how something might happen or how things work changes based on what you are experiencing physically and emotionally right now.

When people come to you, convinced a body part isn't working or is broken in some way, what do you think they experience as they move through their day? And if you at some point told them that picking things up a certain way is bad for their backs, what do you think that does to their mindset around bending? Things will feel harder, less doable, and people will move through the world more cautiously.

When language is used to separate the body from the self, it makes physical tasks during daily routines less connected. People change how they move to reflect their beliefs about what their body is capable of and whether they feel strong and supple.

Embodiment is the connection between the mind and the body. The physical and emotional self become one, and there is no separation or "me versus that body part." You are you.

There is a concept in meditation called open monitoring, which we will discuss in more detail in Chapter 4. It means to observe without judgment, and is an excellent practice for helping people reconnect to their bodies. Below are exercises that use the concepts from open monitoring to teach people how to establish body awareness and shift their mindset, narrowing the chasm between the mind and the body.

Chapter 1

Exercise
Open-monitoring sitting

Come into a comfortable seated position, either on a chair or on the floor. Set a timer for 3 minutes. Close your eyes and begin scanning your body, starting with the toes. As you scan each body part, take a moment to say to yourself, "I feel my feet," "I feel my ankles," "I feel my shins," working your way up the body. Go slowly, and really take the time to feel each part of yourself. As you move through the body, observe how each part feels, without judgment. It can help to imagine the body part in your mind's eye as you are feeling it. Where is it located? How is it positioned?

When the timer goes off, open your eyes, and take a brief moment to observe how you feel mentally. Make a note of it either in a notebook or in your phone. Do you feel calmer or a little more relaxed? Or maybe you feel a little more connected? If you don't feel any change at all, that's okay. Note that, too.

If you aren't used to teaching open monitoring exercises, spend time practicing on yourself. If you struggle with focusing or not judging, as you practice it will get easier. Personal practice also creates the ability to empathize when people struggle. When you observe someone struggling with the same things you have struggled with, it gives you insight into what might help them.

Sitting isn't the new smoking, but maybe lack of daily movement is

One of the headlines that has floated around in recent years is "sitting is the new smoking," causing office workers to embrace standing desks, only for those same office workers to feel confused when new aches crop up from standing all day.

Think for a minute about how you describe what's happening in your life. You may be reaching for a goal, or moving temporarily backward, or in a place of transition. These words, "reaching," "moving," and "transition," all imply physical movement. It's not moving that's dangerous, personally, professionally, or emotionally.

It shouldn't be surprising, then, that the act of sitting isn't bad or unhealthy. In fact, our hips are well designed for sitting – on the ground or on low items, like tree stumps. It's the act of sitting for long periods, stationary, that poses a problem.

Even sitting on the ground – a great position to be in if you have built up the flexibility for it – is only comfortable for so long. As a result, people naturally shift every few minutes, altering their position slightly. Shifting can be as simple as moving from one hip to the other, or it can mean bending one knee up, or bending both knees. The point is that the position people adopt to do specific tasks isn't permanent. It's a state of transition.

I am sitting on the floor, leaning against a wall as I type this. My legs started off long in front of me. They are currently bent so I am sitting cross-legged. My eyes move away from the computer screen and off into the gardens in the distance every so often. My position isn't permanent, which means the way gravity is acting upon my body is constantly changing.

If you work with people who work in office settings, instead of asking them to adopt a specific posture position, ask them to set a timer to go off every 30 minutes. When the timer goes off, ask them to switch positions for a moment. They can reach their arms overhead, stretch their hands to the floor, shift their hips from side to side, or simply nod their head up and down or shake their head from side to side. Invite people to allow themselves a moment to connect with their physical body and chase comfort, not a postural ideal.

I am not suggesting people shouldn't be able to be still. Everyone should be able to rest and relax, but, as a yoga teacher once said to me, "You grow into the position in which you spend the most time." When people spend most of their days sitting, with their arms bent in front of them and their eyes straight ahead, or standing, with their arms in front of them, elbows bent, and their eyes straight ahead scanning the width of a screen, is it any surprise that any movement outside of that is foreign? Or that their back/neck/shoulders/feet ache?

And if people do exercise regularly, which is extremely positive for physical and emotional well-being, that's wonderful, but it's not enough to counteract remaining in the same position for several hours at a time. Planned exercise or sessions with you is different from gentle movement regularly throughout the day. Again, it doesn't take much – just shifting positions occasionally, standing up or sitting down periodically, reaching the arms overhead or behind the body once in a while. These little things can make a big difference in how people feel. But, first, people need to become aware of their normal position. Ask people what they notice. Where is their weight in their feet? What direction do their hands face? How do they lift the leg? Awareness takes practice; instead of always telling people how to move their bodies, ask what they observe and give them the time they need to reflect and answer.

Exercise
Awareness in standing

Come into a standing position. How are you standing? What do you feel?

Shift your weight from side to side. Is one side easier than the other? Notice that, if so.

Now shift your weight forward and back. How does that feel? When you are done shifting, where does your weight naturally settle?

Now, lift one heel up, set it down, and lift the other heel up and set it down. Repeat this five times per side.

Bend your knees a little bit, like you are sinking into the ground, and then straighten your knees. Repeat five times.

Finally, look up towards the ceiling and down towards the floor. Repeat this five times.

When you're finished, take a moment to observe how you are standing now. Has anything changed?

Exercise
Awareness in sitting

Sit on a firm surface so your feet can touch the floor. Set yourself up so you can feel your sitting bones, the two bones at the bottom of the pelvis, against the surface you are sitting on. (No need to move any flesh out of the way. Simply wiggle around until you begin to feel those two points.)

Observe the weight of your feet against the floor. Can you feel how they are resting? Now, observe the weight of the pelvis against the surface you are sitting on. Are you able to sense how it rests on the surface?

Check your jaw and your shoulders. Do they feel tight or like they are clenched or elevated? If so, take an exhale and see if you can allow both to loosen with the exhale.

Rock your pelvis forward, so you roll in front of your sitting bones a little bit, and then rock it backward so you're behind your sitting bones a little bit. Do this five times, resting on your sitting bones after the last one.

Rock slightly from side to side, shifting from one sitting bone to the other, five times per side. Feel how the weight shifts onto each foot and onto each hip. Does one side feel more connected than the other? Or do they feel balanced?

Take a moment to observe the sense of yourself against your seat (Figure 1.3). Do you feel any different?

Chapter 1

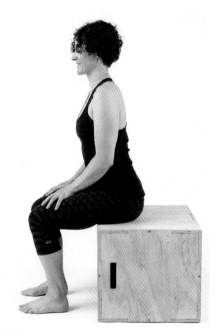

Figure 1.3

Exercise

Awareness in walking

Go for a 10-minute walk. Observe the following areas:

Head position. Do you look down towards the ground, your feet, or your phone, or are your eyes looking up and out?

Torso movement. How does your torso move when you walk? Does your torso stay in front of your hips or behind your hips when you walk? Does it rotate?

The action of the feet. What do they do when you walk? Do your toes turn out or in? Do you feel like your feet stay close to the ground or can you feel they move away from the ground? Is your walking stance narrow or wide? Does one side feel heavier than the other?

Arm movement. Are you usually carrying something or holding something, so your arms are restricted? Or are your arms free to move? If your arms are usually free to move can you feel them swinging easily with each step? Do the arms swing equally?

Pelvis position. Does it rotate forward and back? Does it rock side to side? Does it stay completely still?

These exercises are meant to improve observational skills regarding the physical self. The goal is to invite curiosity, almost like you are exploring these basic everyday movements for the first time. Remember, there is no right or wrong way to perform these basic skills. It could be argued that the fact that your clients and students are successfully moving around and getting through the day means they move just fine. The point is to create a deeper sense of awareness and create a growth mindset, improving self-agency and inviting people to observe, tapping into their connection with their bodies.

References

References

Alhusban RY (2019) Changed body image as perceived by Jordanian women undergoing breast cancer treatment. Asian Pacific Journal of Cancer Prevention 20 (3) 767–773.

Begin C, Turcotte O, and Rodrigue C (2019) Psychosocial factors underlying symptoms of muscle dysmorphia in a non-clinical sample of men. Psychiatry Research 272 319–325.

Bjornsson AS, Didie ER, and Phillips KA (2010) Body dysmorphic disorder. Dialogs in Clinical Neuroscience 12 (2) 221–232.

Citko A, Gorski S, Marcinowicz L, and Gorska A (2018) Sedentary lifestyle and nonspecific low back pain in medical personnel in North-East Poland. Biomedical Research International Article ID 1965807.

da Silva RM, Bezerra MA, Santos-deAraujo AD, de Paula Gomez CAF, da Silva Souza C, de Souza

Matias PHVA, and Dibai-Filho AV (2018) Inactive individuals with chronic neck pain have changes in range of motion and functional performance of the shoulder. Physiotherapy Research International 23 (4) 1,211–1,259.

Dutt-Mazumder A, Rand TJ, Mukherjee M, and Newell KM (2018) Scaling oscillatory platform frequency reveals recurrence of intermittent postural attractor states. Scientific Reports 8 (1) 11,580.

Dweck CS (2006) Mindset: The new psychology of success. New York, NY: Random House.

Ehlers NM, Nielsen CV, and Bjerrum MB (2018) Experiences of older adults after hip fracture: An integrative review. Rehabilitation Nursing 43 (5) 255–266.

Gordon BR, McDowell CP, Lyons M, and Herring MP (2017) The effects of resistance exercise training on anxiety: A meta-analysis and meta-regression analysis of randomized controlled trials. Sports Medicine 47 (12) 2,521–2,532.

Holmes NP and Spence C (2004) The body schema and the multisensory representation(s) of peripersonal space. Cognitive Processing [Electronic] 5 (2) 94–105. Available: https://www.ncbi.nlm.nih.gov/pmc/articles/PMC1350799/

Irvine KR, McCarty K, McKenzie KJ, Pollet TV, Cornelissen KK, Tovee MJ, and Cornelissen PL (2019) Distorted body image influences body schema in individuals with negative bodily attitudes. Neuropsychologia 122 38–50.

Mosconi MW, Mohanty S, and Sweeney JA (2015) Feedforward and feedback motor control abnormalities implicate cerebellar dysfunctions in autism spectrum disorder. The Journal of Neuroscience [Electronic] 35 (5) 2,015–2,025. Available: https://www.ncbi.nlm.nih.gov/pmc/articles/PMC4315832/

Murrie VL, Dixon AK, Hollingworth W, Wilson H, and Doyle TA (2003) Lumbar lordosis: Study of patients with and without low back pain. Clinical Anatomy 16 (2) 144–147.

Nakipoglu GF, Karagoz A, and Ozgirgin N (2008) The biomechanics of the lumbosacral region in acute and chronic low back pain patients. Pain Physician 11 (4) 505–511.

Ng B (2018) The neuroscience of growth mindset and intrinsic motivation. Brain Sciences 8 (2) 20.

Nourbakhsh MR and Arab AM (2002) Relationship between mechanical factors and incidence of low back pain. Journal of Orthopedic Sports Physical Therapy 32 (9) 447–460.

Purcell JB, Winter SR, Breslin CCM, White NC, Lowe MR, and Branch Coslett H (2018) Implicit mental motor imagery task demonstrates a distortion of the body schema in patients with eating disorders. Journal of International Neuropsychology and Sociology 24 (7) 715–723.

Purves D, Augustine GJ, Fitzpatrick D, Katz LC, LaMantia A-S, McNamara JO, and Williams SM (2001) Neuroscience, 2nd edn. Sunderland, MA: Sinauer Associates, Inc.

Ravat S, Olivier B, Gillow N, and Lewis F (2019) Laterality judgement performance between people with chronic pain and pain-free individuals. A systematic review and meta-analysis. Physiotherapy Theory and Practice 1–21.

Shefer S, Gordon C, Avraham KB, and Mintz M (2014) Balance deficit enhances anxiety and balance training decreases anxiety in vestibular mutant mice. Behavioral Brain Research [Electronic] 276. Available: http://kbalab.com/ wp-content/uploads/2012/05/Shefer-et-al_2014.pdf.

Tavares C, Salvi CS, Nisihara R, and Skare T (2018) Low back pain in Brazilian medical students: A cross-sectional study in 629 individuals. Clinical Rheumatology 38 (3) 939–942.

Wirth B, Potthoff T, Rosser S, Humphreys BK, and de Bruin ED (2018) Physical risk factors for adolescent neck and mid back pain: A systematic review. Chiropractic and Manual Therapy [Electronic] 26 (36) 1–10. Available: https://www.ncbi.nlm.nih.gov/pmc/articles/PMC6151922/

Case study

For a long time I worked with a young woman who had been an impressive athlete during high school and college. Her athletic career had resulted in multiple shoulder surgeries, a knee surgery, and low back pain. She was hypermobile, but also hyper-aware, and the pain had significantly decreased her activity level. Though she was only in her late twenties, she said she felt like an 80-year-old woman, scared to pick things up because of the pain she knew she would feel in her back. Fitness classes and yoga made her pain worse, and even though she did her physical therapy exercises diligently, she was frustrated by her discomfort and lack of strength.

A quick assessment of watching her move showed me that while her gross motor patterns were pretty and fluid, her spine remained rigid. She moved around her spine, rather than letting her spine be part of the movement.

This isn't an uncommon strategy. In a small study performed by Seay et al. (2016) subjects with chronic non-specific low back pain and a control group without low back pain were asked to pick up a box from the table beside them and place it down to the floor, a set of movements requiring rotation to get the box from the table and bending to set the box down (the box weighed about 10 kg (23 lb). Subjects with low back pain performed the task using entirely their arms, keeping their backs rigid and still while the control group had less spinal rigidity, allowing their spines to flex, rotate, and extend to while picking up the boxes.

I began by using breath to improve flexion and lateral expansion through her thoracic spine. I also taught her how to move the ribs into a more expiratory position. Once she understood the sensation of the movement, I incorporated isometric holds in a variety of positions, focusing on maintaining rib position. She had a strong bias toward an inspiratory rib position, or ribs flaring forward, which disconnected her from her torso.

When she came in six weeks later (which was how often I saw her), she was carrying herself differently. Her spine was less stiff and her back pain was better. I slowly built more awareness each time I saw her, re-mapping her internal image of her body and where it was in space by using the sensation of work in her abdominals and exercises on the floor to help her feel different parts of her body. By the time she accepted a post-doctorate position out of the country, she had gone for a backpacking trip, was taking yoga classes regularly, and no longer felt like she was going to break. Awareness comes in many different forms; sometimes using the sensation of work in the muscles is the most appropriate choice, but as you will see in subsequent chapters, there are many options when it comes to helping people improve kinesthetic awareness and body confidence.

Where is your body located in space? If I asked you to create a diagram of the area between your shoulder blades, would you be able to conjure up a clear image of the space between your scapulae and what that portion of your back looks like and feels like?

Creating a clear internal image of the body translates to the ability to use the area in an integrated way during movement. Many people beginning their movement journey are disconnected from their bodies. They can't feel various parts of themselves, let alone sense how these foreign body parts contribute to movement. Creating a mindful connection with the body helps the student take ownership of the physical self and makes all aspects of movement training more meaningful.

The disconnect between mind and body isn't specific to sedentary individuals. Individuals who spend time attending group classes or are used to taking instruction on how to move can create strong movement habits and biases, reducing their ability to feel and consciously control different parts of their body. Think of it this way: if you are

continued

always being told how to move your body, it takes away personal choice or a feeling of autonomy by eliminating the opportunity to question, "What feels good? What feels easy? What feels hard? What feels interesting?" Introducing opportunities for students to choose how to move and encouraging students to try different ways of moving improves body schema, proprioception, and increases the mind–body connection.

Proprioception is a sense everyone has that enables them to know, unconsciously, where the body is in space and how it relates to the environment around it.

Kinesthetic awareness refers specifically to an individual's conscious awareness of their body and where it is in relation to things.

If you catch your foot on a curb and quickly right yourself without thinking about it, that's proprioception. If I were to ask you to describe, in detail, how you coordinated your legs to catch yourself so you didn't fall, that's kinesthesia. Both are important, and kinesthesia informs proprioception, but proprioception is a sense, like vision and hearing, that's always thrumming beneath the surface to keep you moving through the world as safely and efficiently as possible.

Both proprioception and kinesthesia can be distorted by things like injuries, trauma, and habitual patterns. Developing these two connected senses requires understanding how they work and how to apply the appropriate technique for the person in front of you.

Improving body awareness can have a profound impact on how your students experience the world and their sense of security in their body. Looking at this another way, if you take the time to teach someone how the body moves and how to explore ways to enhance the ability to feel different parts of the physical body, you are empowering the student to take ownership of the body they possess. We all have the ability to learn; when a person begins improving their body awareness, they are taking the first step to acknowledging that they have the ability to feel more connected to the physical self. This sense of feeling ultimately leads to a greater sense of control over the body and how it's used.

As you move through the next chapters, you will be taken on a journey through exercises and drills that use the concepts of proprioception and kinesthesia to create a deeper awareness of specific parts of the body. Remember, the goal isn't to judge the person you are teaching; rather, it's to look for habits and biases and offer suggestions, inviting curiosity to create a sense of efficiency, ease, and strength.

Imagine there is a glass sitting to your right that you want to pick up. Your ability to reach your right hand the appropriate distance, not knock the glass over, and use the right amount of force to pick the glass up so it doesn't drop is proprioception. Proprioception is a complex interaction of stimuli from the nervous system that is interpreted by the brain, resulting in efferent signals telling the muscles what to do so you can pick up the glass easily. We all rely on proprioception to get through our day without falling or misjudging how hard we need to pull to open the door.

Proprioception is defined as an unconscious perception of movement and spatial orientation that comes from signals in the body. These signals, or stimuli, are detected by nerves and interpreted at the level of the spinal cord or brain, depending on the circumstance. If you pick up a scalding pan accidentally, there will be a reflex reaction to drop the pan. This happens so quickly, the information regarding the temperature of the pan or the position of the hands and fingers doesn't have time to register in the brain before it is dropped (Lorenz et al. 2011; Aman et al. 2014).

When you are picking up the glass in the example above, it's a slower action. The brain has time to interpret arm and hand position and determine the appropriate motor output.

The neuromuscular system (basically, the brain, spinal cord, and the muscles) produce movement by conversing about things like current body position, how tired you are, and how tight/strong/sore you are (Hassan et al. 2000). The central nervous system (CNS) is comprised of the brain and spinal cord. It assesses available movement options via information from one of the branches of the peripheral nervous system (PNS), the afferent or sensory branch.

The afferent nervous system shares information with the CNS about things like pressure on the skin, how much stretch a certain muscle is under, how much force a muscle is generating, the position of the joints, or whether something is painful.

Let's say you are on a couch with your legs up on the back cushions, your knees bent and to the left, your right ankle crossed over the left, and you decide you want to get up. How would you do it?

Fortunately, you don't need to consciously think about it because your CNS would use the information it has based on the angles of your joints, how you've gotten up in the past, and whether there's any stretch/strain/pain in any parts of your body that would affect how you can easily get up off of the couch. Your brain would send motor neurons to the musculoskeletal system to coordinate the action of the joints and activate the appropriate muscles and you would stand up.

You probably guessed I was the one in the precarious arrangement on the couch. I just stood up, and it turns out I accomplished the movement by swinging my right leg to the side of the couch so I could stand on my right foot to balance. My left foot followed and I stood up. I tried it again, and the second time I pushed off the side of the couch with my left arm to propel myself sideways. Your nervous system chooses the most efficient way to accomplish the task

given the information it has. Your habitual movement patterns influence the nervous system and its determination of how to perform tasks like getting up off of the couch quickly and easily. If you always move the same way to get up or down, your nervous system will "forget" there are other ways to do it, which means that sometimes there are more efficient ways of doing exactly the same thing. It just requires a bit more conscious thought.

My ability to discern how I performed the movement and my perception of the position of my body and limbs is my kinesthetic awareness. Kinesthesia, remember, happens consciously while proprioception occurs unconsciously (Riemann & Lephart 2002).

Proprioception, along with the eyes and inner ear, also contributes to your sense of stability (Longo & Haggard 2010). If you were to stand up right now and close your eyes, hopefully you wouldn't tip over, but your postural sway might increase. Postural sway is the gentle movement that occurs when you stand as your brain works on maintaining your balance. You are never perfectly still when you stand; the mechanoreceptors in your ankles and feet are constantly sending information about the location of your joints, working with your visual and vestibular system to act as your internal global positioning system (GPS). When you remove one sense, such as your eyes, you still have proprioception and your inner ears to keep you upright.

Proprioception, like all of our senses, can be developed with practice. Often students who are new to a movement setting haven't challenged their proprioception or worked to develop it for a long time, perhaps for years. This means that when they perform a balance task, change direction, or estimate how much force is needed to pick up an object, their accuracy of how to perform these challenges won't be finely tuned. If you treat proprioception like a skill and choose exercises to enhance proprioception, it will improve, along with strength, mobility, and coordination.

Improving proprioception can improve a person's sense of stability and confidence, and decrease anxiety, all important measures of quality of life: as I mentioned previously, the proprioceptive information the nervous system sends to the brain prevents falling. In fact, proprioceptive information is often relayed faster than visual information, which means one aspect to a fall-prevention program should be proprioceptive training (Cameron et al. 2014). Placing people in safe situations where they can take the time to figure out where the body is in relation to the ground and giving them time to generate the appropriate sequence of movements to resist gravity so they can effectively return to a stable position is one way to incorporate more complex proprioceptive training.

One of the other things proprioception does is help people determine how much force is needed to perform a certain task. Let's say someone tells you the box on the floor is filled with books and it needs to be moved. Based on how much you think a book weighs, the size of the box, and your ability to generate force, you will be able to accurately predict how much strength you need to lift it. Past experience, your current physical abilities, and the information you take in based on your visual assessment enable you to successfully lift an object that's different from any other object you've ever lifted, since no two boxes of books are exactly the same.

If, on the other hand, the box was actually filled with down pillows, when you go to lift the box you might find yourself thrown off balance because it's lighter than you expected. You inaccurately predicted the amount of force needed and your nervous system responded by sending lots of impulses to the muscles. Your nervous system responds by quickly righting you, adjusting to the feedback recovered from the afferent nervous system.

How accurately and quickly someone can make these types of adjustments is influenced by internal body image, available strength due to muscle size, and the angle of the joints when the person is picking up the box. If you had very little experience picking up boxes of varying weights, it would be more difficult for you to adapt to the unexpectedly light box. If, however, you spent lots of time lifting boxes, your nervous system would draw from past experience and quickly adjust force and balance, allowing you to recalibrate without falling over.

Remember when we discussed body schema in Chapter 1? The accuracy of your body schema is determined largely by your proprioception. Your body schema is what allows you to navigate the world without running into things, so you can intuitively know whether you can squeeze through a narrow space, or duck under an object and not hit your head (D'Angelo et al. 2018). Your body schema plays an important role in integrating senses such as touch and proprioception, affecting the relationship of the body and its interaction with the environment (Morasso et al. 2015).

There are a number of things that affect body schema, including how much time you spend using a body part and the way in which you use that specific body part.

Let's say you are working with a student who has spent years keeping their shoulders down and back. When they imagine their shoulders, they imagine they are away from the ears and back, behind the hips. This makes their image of the shoulders in relation to the actual size of their shoulders small or less present. If you had the student shift the shoulders forward and asked what that felt like, they may respond that it feels strange or like they are slouching. The movement habits people adopt can result in a rigid internal sense of a physical area if they never practice moving differently.

In this example, simply asking the person to move the shoulders up and down will begin recreating the internal image of the shoulder. Feeling how the shoulder moves reminds the student that the shoulder can move many different ways. It's not just a fixed object that stays in one position. Often, the simple act of moving the shoulder will begin to decrease the sensation of stiffness or pain. The more of yourself you can feel, the more of yourself you will use, creating more fluidity and coordination while moving through life.

Exercise
Altering the perception of the arm

Come into a seated position with your arms by your side and your feet flat on the floor. Think about the outlines of your arms. How long are they? Do they feel the same length?

Now, imagine your left arm is holding a yardstick, the end of which is resting against the floor. Point the yardstick up toward the wall in front of you. Repeat the movement six times, each time reaching the imaginary yardstick toward the wall as much as you can.

Raise your right arm up toward the wall in front of you, without your imaginary yardstick, reaching the hand toward the wall. Repeat six times.

Rest your hands by your sides. Imagine the outlines of your arms. Does one feel longer than the other?

There is a pretty good chance you felt like your left arm was longer than the right by the end of the exercise above. That's because when you use a tool or an implement, your brain adopts that item into your schema – the item becomes a part of you. You "know" how much space your limb takes up with the tool and how your limb holding the tool will interact with your surrounding environment (Martel et al. 2016).

Many of our students and clients walk around with cell phones in their hands or with their heads looking down at screens. This can lead to the adoption of certain habitual movement patterns, like moving the arm as though the phone is still attached to it. It can also lead to the formation of specific habits like always walking with the head and eyes looking downwards or an arm that doesn't swing because it's become accustomed to holding a specific tool.

An easy way to see someone's preferred habits is to observe students walking. In what direction are the eyes oriented? Do the arms swing? Does the thoracic spine rotate? Does the pelvis rotate? Does one arm look heavy, like it's used to holding up a purse or a phone?

This constant honing and fine tuning the nervous system does with the body and its environment can also be altered by previous physical experiences. For instance, people who have lost quite a bit of weight in a short amount of time may have an altered internal image of what they look like. Their brain remembers the amount of space they used to take up, so often their movements still reflect their heavier selves. They may walk differently, with their legs wide set for balance, or they may take a wide berth around objects, even though they take up less room than they used to. Individuals with eating disorders such as anorexia also have an altered internal map of what their bodies look like, believing they, too, take up more space than they actually do (Riva 2014). In both cases, the perception of the body in space and the reality of the body in space conflict, affecting motor patterns. When working with these individuals, it's important to be sensitive to their beliefs, while still creating opportunities for them to re-create a more accurate representation of self.

The brain is constantly integrating sensory information to create an accurate representation of the experience of the body; however, this representation, or image, is highly adaptable and can be altered by perception (Saloman et al. 2016).

Chapter 2

Case study

I trained a man for several years who had lost 39 kg (85 lb) years before we started working together. He was in his seventies when he began training with me. He stood back in his heels, belly forward, as though he were still accommodating the extra weight. He walked with a wider step, which was necessary when he was heavier, but not necessary in his smaller body.

As I slowly encouraged him to shift his weight to different places, he told me every time he looked in the mirror he was still surprised at this new, smaller version of himself. He didn't fully believe that he took up so much less space. He embodied a much larger man, and as a result he moved with the slowness and heaviness of someone with a larger body.

As we worked together, he slowly learned he didn't need to move with the same heaviness. He became a little more comfortable balancing and maneuvering with his smaller frame, though I don't think he ever fully took ownership of his "new" body. He held on to an older image, resistant to altering his self-perception.

One of the easiest ways to begin improving internal image is through touch, either using self-touch or the touch of someone else. Touch stimulates the sensory receptors in the skin that detect changes in pressure (Abrairaa & Ginty 2013). These changes in pressure are noted by the brain and provide the sensory nervous system with information about the size and location of the area that is being touched. The brain is then able to incorporate this new information about the body into its framework for movement.

This is one of the reasons foam rolling and other self-massage tools may be effective at temporarily reducing the sensation of stiffness (MacGregor et al. 2018). The pressure from the object against the skin stimulates mechanoreceptors responsible for things like stretch and detection of force. The student's experience of the body changes because of the sensory feedback and the student feels more flexible for a short period of time. This creates a window of opportunity for the student to use the "new," more full range of motion in movement, reinforcing the range of motion through strength and mobility.

Of course, like with most things related to the body and sensation, there are other inputs occurring, influencing a person's experience and perception. In the cells are specialized peripheral sensory neurons called nociceptors. Nociceptors detect sensations like extreme pressure and temperature that could be potentially damaging to the organism. When a student places the weight of their leg on a foam roller, the strong sensation they feel could be interpreted as pain.

Pain is defined as a complex interplay between factors such as unpleasant sensory, cognitive, or emotional experiences caused by tissue damage or perceived tissue damage. It manifests through autonomic, behavioral, and psychological reactions (Dubin & Patapoutian 2010). The perception of pain is highly individualized and subjective. Nociceptors detect sensation; how the sensation is interpreted varies from person to person.

Let's say you grabbed a hot pan again, like in the example earlier (you forgot it was hot). The nociceptors in your skin would loudly inform you there has been a significant, potentially damaging change in temperature at the site of your hand. Your nervous system would send information to the hand via the motor neurons to drop the pan (again).

Instead of a hot pan, pretend you reach down to pick up a weight that's on the right side of your body with your right hand. You have been told picking up heavy objects may be bad for your back and your shoulder. As you pick up the weight, you feel sensation through your arm. You determine the sensation you are feeling is pain.

continued

Case study *continued*

If I picked up the same weight, but I believe picking up the weight is going to strengthen my tissues, I may also feel a sensation in my arm, but I determine the sensation is the sensation of my arm adjusting to how to hold the weight. As a result, I will have a different relationship with what I am experiencing.

The pain a student feels when they place pressure on their thigh with a foam roller increases the pressure pain threshold (Aboodarda et al. 2015). This means that immediately following time spent using the foam roller on the quadriceps, the student will be able to place more pressure on their thigh with less sensitivity. Why this works is unclear, though evidence suggests foam rolling improves arterial dilation and vascular plasticity. It also reduces the sensation of fatigue, increases range of motion, and improves tissue recovery when exercise-induced muscular soreness is present. It may even improve neuromuscular efficiency, making massage tools a potentially worthwhile aid for recovery and during a student's warm-up.

The other reason foam rolling may work is that applying pressure to an area that feels painful seems to inhibit the perception of pain throughout the entire body, not just in the area where the pressure is applied. So, rolling out a painful quadriceps muscle might make an achy shoulder feel better, even though no pressure has been applied to the shoulder. It's as though the pressure creates a relaxation response, down-regulating the sympathetic nervous system. Using massage tools for people who are prone to stiffness or who have fear around movement can create an opportunity for more movement. It's easier to move when things feel less stiff and don't hurt; applying pressure also increases awareness of the body part where pressure was applied, possibly making it easier to integrate the area into skills or exercises (hence, an increase in neuromuscular efficiency).

You can implement the concepts of applying pressure even if you don't have a foam roller or ball available. Two easy places to apply pressure are the hands and the feet; this can reap big benefits in terms of the student's ability to feel and use those areas.

Exercise

Hand-pressure awareness

Take a moment to notice your hands and how they feel. How big do they feel? How much space do they take up?

Now, turn your right palm over so it's facing the ceiling. Take your left thumb to the center of the right palm and wrap the other fingers around the back of the hand. Press your left thumb into the center of the palm and use the thumb to keep gentle pressure on the hand as you move the left thumb all of the way out to the end of the right pinkie finger, maintaining consistent pressure. Take the left thumb back to the center of the right palm and repeat this three times. Then, starting with your left thumb in the center of the right palm, do the same thing with the fourth finger of the right hand, the middle finger, the index finger, and the thumb (you may have to angle your right hand in to get to the thumb) (Figure 2.1).

Once you have finished, pause with your hands by your side. Do your hands feel different from each other? Which hand feels larger?

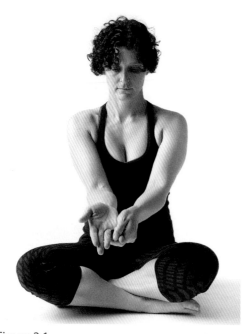

Figure 2.1

Exercise
Foot-sensation awareness

Come into a seated position on a chair with your feet flat on the floor under your knees. Cross your right ankle over your left knee, as though you were putting a sock on your right foot.

Take your right hand on top of the right foot, holding it lightly. Use the left thumb and index finger to get a hold of the right pinkie toe. Pull the pinkie toe out, away from the foot, and back, toward the right heel. It's like you are reaching it forward and then pulling it back.

Do this three or four times and then move on to the fourth toe, performing the same movement three or four times before moving on to the third toe, eventually doing all of the toes.

Now, place the left pinkie finger between the right fourth toe and pinkie toe and the left ring finger between the fourth toe and the third toe, and the middle finger between the right third

toe and second toe and the left index finger between the right second toe and big toe. You will have created toe spreaders for your right foot with your left fingers.

Use the left hand to gently move the right foot up and down, side to side, and in a circle (Figure 2.2). Remove your left fingers from between the right toes. How does your right foot feel compared to your left foot?

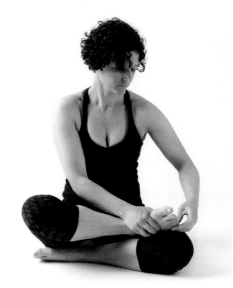

Figure 2.2

Using touch, either through massage, self-massage, or with a tool such as a foam roller, provides a gateway to improved proprioception. The key to making this newfound awareness last is to use the body afterward in new ways, creating an imprint of how the body maneuvers itself through space.

Another form of touch that can be used to improve proprioception is tapping the skin using the fingers, tapping a body part against the floor, or having a tool vibrate against the skin. If the brain is healthy and no neurological disease is present, the touch input will stimulate the afferent nervous system, reinforcing a sense of body ownership (Kilteni & Ehrsson 2017). Body ownership results in more coordinated and efficient movement. It also results in the student feeling more secure during movement.

A form of feedback that is similar to tapping, but done using a machine that vibrates, is whole body vibration (WBV) therapy. WBV therapy has been found to decrease the perception of soreness that occurs from exercise, improve spinal proprioception, and help with the management of pain related to knee osteoarthritis (Iodice et al. 2018; Chow et al. 2018; Ferreira et al. 2018). Vibration and tapping are both inputs to the afferent nervous system that result in a neurological – and maybe even physical – response. Using tools like the Power Plate® or Galileo®, machines that vibrate at low frequencies, can be useful when working with students in a post-rehabilitation setting or with students who struggle with feeling stable or grounded.

Tapping the fingers on the body can also down-regulate the nervous system, suppressing the stress response (Stears et al. 2017). The autonomic nervous system is split into two branches: the parasympathetic nervous system and the sympathetic nervous system. The parasympathetic nervous system is active during periods of rest, digestion, and relaxation. The sympathetic nervous system is considered the fight-or-flight nervous system, though research suggests an individual's response to stress is influenced by mindset: does the person view stressors as a challenge, or is stress viewed as something to be avoided at all costs (Horiuchi et al. 2018)? If stress is viewed as potentially threatening and to be avoided, their physiological response will differ from someone who views stress as a challenge, which will be reflected in heart rate, respiration rate, breathing strategy, and muscle tone.

The two branches of the autonomic nervous system complement each other quite well. During different periods of the day, one branch will be more active than the other, because after a large meal it's natural for the parasympathetic nervous system to kick into high gear so you can rest and digest, just like it's natural for the sympathetic nervous system to activate when you are about to give a lecture to a room full of people. Feeling appropriately stimulated or appropriately restful creates a balanced way of being.

Occasionally, people experience more sympathetic nervous system activity than is actually necessary, which can lead to irritability, anxiety, and the general feeling of chronic stress. A regular dose of stress is actually good. From a physiological perspective, stress in the form of load stimulates the cells to respond by making the tissues (muscles, bones, tendons) stronger (Hernandez & Kravitz n.d.). Stress promotes growth and strength, but too much stress before the system is adequately prepared to handle it can cause depletion and injury or illness. When you begin lifting weights or start practicing a new movement modality, for instance, the tissues adapt to the demands imposed upon them. However, if you do the exact same exercise or movement daily, in exactly the same way without any variation, the tissues don't have an opportunity to recover. The muscles and joints may become achy and chronically sore. Designing an effective movement program takes into account both stress and rest, leading to strength. Resilience and adaptation occur in the sweet spot between stress and rest.

An effective way to regulate sympathetic nervous system activity in chronically stressed individuals is through movement of all kinds, including general exercise. Feelings of anxiety and depression, which often accompany chronic stress, can also be improved through movement that improves the mind–body connection (Liu et al. 2018). This probably occurs for a number of reasons, one of which is the fact that paying attention to a specific task, such as a movement practice, focuses attention. It's no secret that attention is split these days between different devices, different projects, and trying to lead a balanced life. Daily life can feel overwhelming and lead to a general sense of fatigue. Using mindful movement modalities can cultivate benefits that are similar to what people would get from a meditation practice (Telles et al. 2018; Payne & Crane-Godreau 2013). Tapping is frequently used in mindful movement techniques such as Qi Gong, martial arts, and Feldenkrais Method®, eliciting a mind–body connection and focusing attention prior to more global movement patterns.

Chapter 2

Exercise
Tapping

This can be done either seated or standing. Find a comfortable position. Gently cup your left hand and turn the palm toward the center of your chest. Use your left fingers to tap the center of your chest, moving the hand to tap under the collar bones to the outside of the right shoulder, down the outside of the right arm to the hand, back up the inside of the right arm to the center of the chest (Figure 2.3). Do this two or three times.

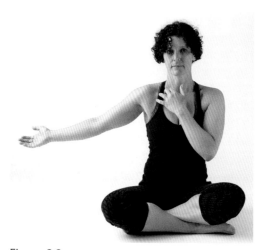

Figure 2.3

Switch hands, doing the same thing with right hand across the chest, down the left arm, and back up the left arm. Pause for a moment when you finish. How do you feel?

Come into a standing position. Make gentle fists with your hands. Begin lightly tapping the two front hip bones with your fists, moving around to the low back and pelvis. You can either keep your hands in fists or open them to slap down the outside of your legs and back up the inside of the legs, tapping the front of the hip bones again when you make your back to the starting position. Do this two or three times. Rest your hands and pause for a moment. How do you feel?

Lift your right heel and let tap against the ground as it lowers down. Feel the echo of the movement up your torso. Lift your left heel and let it tap against the ground as it lowers down. Alternate the heels for about 30 seconds, letting each one tap into the ground and feel how that creates awareness up the heel into the leg.

Once you are finished, take a moment to observe your breath and your body. Note how you feel.

Shaking

Have you ever watched professional basketball players before they take a free throw? Many of them shake their arms before they make the shot. The same is true of Olympic swimmers, divers, and baseball players in the dugout. Shaking is a natural way to "shake off the nerves" before you are about to do something stressful. Shaking discharges physical tension, making the athlete feel calmer and less anxious about whatever they are about to do (Berceli et al. 2014).

Shaking is kind of like a whole body vibration. Since most of us don't have access to vibration plates or vibration units commonly used in WBV therapy, having the ability to create your own vibration through shaking can provide a host of benefits.

Exercise
Shaking

Come into a standing position, with your feet resting comfortably on the floor. If standing is uncomfortable for you, you can do the same exercise seated: there will just be a little less shake.

Begin gently shaking your head from side to side, as though you were a bobblehead doll. Keep everything loose, and keep the movement really small. Perform this for 10 seconds.

Stop shaking the head and begin shaking the arms. I like to imagine I am flicking water off of my hands. Perform this for 10 seconds.

Keep your elbows by your sides and shake out just your hands. Perform this for 10 seconds.

If you are standing, make sure you are near a wall for balance. Lift your left foot and shake your left leg rapidly without losing your balance. Perform this for 10 seconds and switch sides.

Now, let your whole body shake for 10 seconds. When you are finished, hold still for a moment. How do you feel?

Tapping and shaking can be performed as part of a warm-up to a class or as a way to connect with a specific body part. I frequently use foot tapping or shaking directly before teaching an exercise that emphasizes the feet and how they interact with the ground. I also find shaking to be particularly effective for dissipating excess tension prior to teaching breathing exercises or relaxation techniques.

Case study

When Alex first came in to see me, his movements were stiff and a bit awkward. He was struggling with hamstring tendinosis in both legs and the occasional bout of back pain. Tendinosis occurs when the tendon's collagen degenerates because of chronic overuse. It causes pain, decreases strength and flexibility, and affects function (Bass 2012). Alex basically had chronic hamstring pain that was impacting his quality of life.

When I would have Alex perform balance-type activities, such as balancing on his right leg as he lifted his left leg, his hands would stiffen even more, giving him a sense of stability. This isn't uncommon. When people have chronic pain or feel as though they lack strength or stability, they will often create the feeling of stability by clenching other areas. While this can be an effective way to maintain balance, the act of lifting one leg off of the ground doesn't require high amounts of effort. In many cases, individuals who use a clenching strategy prior to movement don't feel themselves tensing as they do a seemingly unrelated movement, such as lifting a leg.

This was definitely the case for Alex. It wasn't until I drew attention to his hands that he could feel them tensing. However, he wasn't sure how to change the behavior by making them less tense. I began having Alex shake his hands and arms out in between sets of balance exercises to improve his awareness of his hands and how he held them. Over time, he learned to feel when he was clenching his hands unnecessarily. This translated to an increased awareness of hand clenching throughout the day. He discovered if he found himself clenching, he could shake his arms out and continue working, decreasing his overall tension.

Chapter 2

Force

One final tactic for improving proprioception around the joints is to create force through muscular contraction. This works by creating sensation and drawing conscious awareness to an area.

The sensation that is caused through contraction occurs because of specialized cells called mechanoreceptors. These cells are located in the part of the muscle that detects changes in muscle length and the speed at which a limb changes position. When limb muscles contract, the nervous system sends extra information to the brain about the body position that directly impacts kinesthetic awareness (Proske & Gandevia 2009).

Both ligaments and tendons have elastic properties, but they aren't as elastic as muscle (Petrofsky et al. 2013). Ligaments restrict movement to be within a certain range and are extremely strong, allowing them to control position and movements through the musculoskeletal system (Biewener 2008). Everyone is born with a certain degree of flexibility in the ligaments, otherwise known as laxity. Some people naturally have high degrees of laxity in several joints. These individuals are often called hypermobile. Anywhere from 4% to 13% of the population has generalized joint laxity, another term for individuals with hypermobility who don't have joint pain or discomfort related to their extra flexibility (Simpson 2006).

There is a spectrum of hypermobility, ranging from generalized joint laxity to a collagen disorder called Ehlers-Danlos syndrome (EDS), a syndrome that can affect skin, ligaments, and blood vessels (Nuytinck et al. 2000). Collagen disorders such as EDS are diagnosed by medical professionals and often require being under the care of a medical professional. Benign joint hypermobility is a form of hypermobility that results in joint pain and discomfort. It is a connective tissue disorder that is often considered a milder variant of EDS and is seen in up to 3% of the population (Kumar et al. 2017). Hypermobility in a non-clinical setting is generally tested through the Beighton test, which assesses joint range of motion at a variety of joints, including the fingers, wrists, knees, and elbows (Beighton et al. 2012).

Some people with hypermobility report feeling unstable, as though their arms are going to fall out of their sockets, or their ribs are going to dislocate. I have also had hypermobile clients complain of sensations of tightness and the desire to stretch, despite the fact their joint range of motion exceeds normal ranges. Feeling stable and decreasing the sensation of tightness comes from creating force through contraction as opposed to passively stretching.

Hypermobility can occur in just one joint instead of several joints. Hypermobility is not a disease; in fact, as noted above, in many cases it doesn't cause pain or discomfort. It only becomes an issue when the individual lacks control, strength, and stability at the hypermobile joint.

Injuries can cause hypermobility in other areas as well. Have you ever sprained an ankle? Even after it heals, people report sensations of instability or lack of balance years later (Hubbard & Hicks-Little 2008). One potential cause of chronic ankle instability following an acute ankle sprain is ligaments that don't fully heal. Remember how ligaments are filled with sensory receptors that inform proprioception? When they become overstretched (which is what happens in an ankle sprain), the information the nervous system receives regarding the joint is that it is unstable. Ligaments are naturally stiff structures that aren't meant to stretch excessive amounts. When stress in the form of acute trauma occurs and the ligament exceeds its stretch capacity, perception of the joint is altered, which means proprioception is affected.

The mechanoreceptors that are embedded in ligaments allow you to subconsciously know the position of your joints even when you aren't thinking about them (Dhillon et al. 2012). When there has been damage to a ligament, the information the nervous system receives may be fuzzy. The ability to consciously feel joint position and detect really small changes in position can improve both the conscious (kinesthetic awareness), and the subconscious (proprioceptive) awareness (Konradsen 2002).

Applying force to the joints via muscular contraction benefits kinesthesia and proprioception. Force can be applied both internally, by actively tensing a specific area, or externally, by holding a heavy object. If a student has hypermobility in a specific joint and is receiving information that the joint isn't being held together well because the ligaments aren't stiff, using muscular contractions in the muscles around the hypermobile joint tells the neuromuscular system that the joint is supported; the nervous system responds by creating a sensation of joint stability. Feeling more stable creates a sensation of safety, and feeling safer reduces sensations of anxiety, which improves emotional well-being. When a joint feels more secure, the willingness to move more, in a variety of ways, increases.

Another benefit to having the ability to consciously contract muscles is it makes it easier to feel the opposite of contraction. If you are working with someone who experiences tightness in the neck, for instance, while observing their movements, you may find the student's habit is to keep the shoulders elevated. When you ask the student to relax the shoulders, they don't move. You can ask the student to exaggerate the habit by having them tense the shoulders up by the ears even more than normal. The student will then be able to feel how to perform the opposite action, relaxing the shoulders down. Making the tension seem really, really obvious reminds the brain, "Oh! That's what it feels like to tense a muscle. Relaxation is the opposite feeling." Put more simply: consciously contracting leads to consciously relaxing.

Exercise
Consciously tensing the upper extremity

Come into a seated position, allowing your arms to hang by your sides. Feel the weight of your arms. Take a moment here to breathe, observing the sensation of the arms by your sides.

Make strong fists with your hands, clenching your fists as much as you can for two breaths, and then relaxing. Do this two times.

Now, bend your elbows, and begin clenching the muscles in your upper arms, tightening them for two breaths, and then relaxing (Figure 2.4). Do this two times.

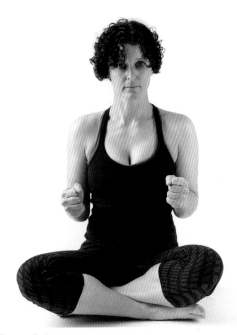

Figure 2.4

Take your arms back by your sides, make fists with your hands, and straighten them out to the sides, making a "T" with the body. Keep them there as you tighten all of the muscles in your arms. Hold it for two breaths and relax. Do this two times.

Rest with your arms by your sides. Feel the weight of your arms. Do they feel heavier? Lighter? The same?

Using techniques such as the one described above can be effective directly before relaxation exercises or before movements that require less tension, such as ground-based work or unloaded transition work.

Chapter 2

Interoception

Interoception is a word that is frequently thrown around with proprioception, despite the fact they are two different things. Interoception is the sense of internal physiological sensations. It is the accurate observation of the physiological senses, which is actually different than spatial awareness, though it has similarities and is influenced by kinesthetic awareness. It's the process of the nervous system sensing, interpreting, and integrating signals originating from within the body, creating a map of the body's inner workings on a conscious and unconscious level (Mehling et al. 2018). Interoception is the ability to observe respiration rate, heart rate, and how you feel internally. Interoception is important because, like kinesthesia, it creates a more complete picture of the physical and emotional state.

For instance, when someone first begins an exercise program they may notice their muscles burn when they try to hold a bent knee position for more than one breath. This is an observation of the interoceptive state.

Interoception can tell you about emotional responses as well. I was in a terrifying car accident a few years ago, one that left a scary impression. As the car that was spinning three lanes away began ping ponging toward me and I maneuvered, trying to change lanes and avoid it, I realized I wasn't going to be able to get out of the car's way fast enough.

I don't remember the impact, but as I moved over to the side of the road, I checked myself to make sure I felt okay. I was breathing quickly and my heart was audible in my chest. My interoceptive awareness told me I was feeling stressed, but nothing was damaged.

Both interoception and proprioception are beneficial skills to help people hone. The goal isn't to make students hypervigilant, monitoring their physiological states 24 hours a day. Rather, the goal is to empower students with the tools to check in with their internal sense of self, once in a while, so they can gauge their mental and physical states. We will discuss interoception in more detail in Chapter 3, but, for now, consider that helping students feel more of their bodies and interpret how they physically feel when they experience inputs like touch, force, and vibration can impact more than just their movement experience.

References

Aboodarda SJ, Spence AJ, and Button DC (2015) Pain pressure threshold of a muscle tender spot increases following local and non-local rolling massage. BMC Musculoskeletal Disorders [Electronic] 16 265. Available: https://www.ncbi.nlm.nih.gov/pmc/articles/PMC4587678/.

Abrairaa V and Ginty DD (2013) The sensory neurons of touch. Neuron [Electronic] 79 (4). Available: https://www.ncbi.nlm.nih.gov/pmc/articles/PMC3811145/pdf/nihms 514231. pdf.

Aman JE, Elangovan N, Yeh I-L, and Konczak, J (2014) The effectiveness of proprioceptive training for improving motor function: A systematic review. Frontiers in Human Neuroscience [Electronic] 8 1,075. Available: https://www. ncbi.nlm.nih.gov/pmc/articles/PMC4309156/.

Bass E (2012) Tendinopathy: Why the difference between tendinitis and tendinosis matters. International Journal of Therapeutic Massage & Bodywork 5 (1) 14–17.

Beighton PH, Grahame R, and Bird HA (2012) Assessment of hypermobility, Chapter 2 in Hypermobility of joints, 4th edn. London: Springer-Verlag.

Berceli D, Salmon M, Bonifas R, and Ndefo N (2014) Effects of self-induced unclassified therapeutic tremors on quality of life among non-professional caregivers: A pilot study. Global Advances in Health Medicine 3 (5) 45–48.

Biewener A (2008) Tendons and ligaments: Structure, mechanical behavior and biological function, in Fratzl P (ed.) Collagen. Boston, MA: Springer.

Cameron BD, de la Malla C, and Lopez-Moliner J (2014) The role of differential delays in integrating transient visual and proprioceptive information. Frontiers of Psychology 5 50.

Chow DHK, Lee TY, and Pope MH (2018) Effects of whole body vibration on spinal proprioception in healthy individuals. Work 61 (3) 403–411.

D'Angelo M, di Pellegrino G, Seriani S, Gallina P, and Frassinetti F (2018) The sense of agency shapes body schema and peripersonal space. Nature [Electronic] 8 13,847. Available: https://www.ncbi.nlm.nih.gov/pmc/articles/PMC6138644/pdf/41598_2018_Article_32238.pdf.

Dhillon MS, Bali K, and Prabhakar S (2012) Differences among mechanoreceptors in healthy and injured anterior cruciate ligaments and their clinical importance. Muscles Ligaments and Tendons Journal [Electronic] 2 (1) 38–43. Available: https://www.ncbi.nlm.nih.gov/pmc/articles/PMC3666492/.

Dubin AE and Patapoutian A (2010) Nociceptors: The sensory of the pain pathway. The Journal of Clinical Investigation [Electronic] 120 (11) 3,760–3,772. Available: https://www.ncbi.nlm.nih.gov/pmc/articles/PMC2964977/.

Ferreira RM, Duarte JA, and Goncalves RS (2018) Non-pharmacological and non-surgical interventions to manage patients with knee arthritis: An umbrella review. Acta Reumatologica Portuguesa 43 (3) 182 200.

Hassan BS, Mockett S, and Doherty M (2000) Static postural sway, proprioception, and maximal voluntary quadriceps contraction in patients with knee osteoarthritis and normal control subjects. Annals of the Rheumatic Diseases [Electronic] 60 612–618. Available: https://www.ncbi.nlm.nih.gov/pmc/articles/PMC1753664/pdf/v060p00612.pdf

Hernandez RS and Kravitz L (n.d.) The mystery of skeletal muscle hypertrophy. Available: http://www.unm.edu/~lkravitz/Article%20folder/hypertrophy.html.

Horiuchi S, Tsuda A, Aoki S, Yoneda K, and Sawaguch Y (2018) Coping as a mediator of the relationship between stress mindset and psychological stress response: A pilot study. Psychology Research and Behavior Management [Electronic] 11 47–54. Available: https://www.ncbi.nlm.nih.gov/pmc/articles/PMC5840190/.

Hubbard TJ and Hicks-Little CA (2008) Ankle ligament healing after an acute ankle sprain: An evidence based approach. Journal of Athletic Training [Electronic] 43 (5) 523–529. Available: https://www.ncbi.nlm.nih.gov/pmc/articles/PMC2547872/.

Iodice P, Ripari P, and Pezzulo G (2018) Local high-frequency vibration therapy following eccentric exercises reduces muscle soreness perception and posture alterations in elite athletes. European Journal of Applied Physiology 119 (2) 539–549.

Kilteni K and Ehrsson HH (2017) Body ownership determines the attenuation of self-generated tactile body sensations. Proceedings of the National Academy of Sciences of the United States of America [Electronic] 114 (31) 8,426–8,431. Available: https://www.ncbi.nlm.nih.gov/pmc/articles/PMC5547616/.

Konradsen L (2002) Factors contributing to chronic ankle instability: Kinesthesia and joint position sense. Journal of Athletic Training [Electronic] 37 (4) 381–385. Available: https://www.ncbi.nlm.nih.gov/pmc/articles/PMC164369/.

Kumar B and Lenert P (2017) Joint hypermobility syndrome: Recognizing a commonly overlooked cause of pain. The American Journal of Medicine 130 640-647.

Liu Z, Wu Y, Li L, and Guo X (2018) Functional connectivity within the executive control network mediates the effects of long-term Tai Chi exercises on elders' emotion regulation. Frontiers of Aging in Neuroscience 10 315.

Longo MR and Haggard P (2010) An implicit body representation underlying human position sense. Proceedings of the National Academy of Sciences of the United States of America [Electronic] 107 (26)

11,727–11,732. Available: https://www.pnas.org/content/pnas/107/26/11727.full.pdf.

Lorenz MD, Coates JR, and Kent M (2011) Handbook of veterinary neurology, 5th edn. St. Louis, MO: W.B. Saunders. Available: https://doi.org/10.1016/B978-1-4377-0651-2.10017-7.

MacGregor LJ, Fairweather MM, Bennett RM, and Hunter AM (2018) The effect of foam rolling for three consecutive days on muscular efficiency and range of motion. Sports Medicine-Open [Electronic] 4 26. Available: https://www.ncbi.nlm.nih.gov/pmc/articles/PMC5993692/.

Martel M, Cardinali L, Roy AC, and Farne A. (2016) Tool-use: An open window into bod representation and its plasticity. Cognitive Neuropsychology 33 (1–2) 82–101.

Mehling WE, Acree M, Stewart A, Silas J, and Jones A (2018) The multidimensional assessment of interoceptive awareness, version 2. PLOS One [Electronic]. Available: https://journals.plos.org/plosone/article?id=10.1371/journal.pone.0208034.

Morasso P, Casadio M, Mohan V, Rea F, and Zenzeri J (2015) Revisiting the body-schema concept in the context of whole-body postural-focal dynamics. Frontiers in Human Performance 9 83.

Nuytinck L, Freund M, Lagae L, Pierard GE, Hermanns-Le T, and De Paepe A (2000) Classical Ehlers-Danlos Syndrome caused by a mutation in type I collagen. American Journal of Human Genetics [Electronic] 66 (4) 1,398–1,402. Available: https://www.ncbi.nlm.nih.gov/ pmc/articles/PMC1288203/.

Payne P and Crane-Godreau MA (2013) Meditative movement for depression and anxiety. Frontiers in Psychiatry [Electronic] 4 71. Available: https://www.ncbi.nlm.nih.gov/pmc/articles/PMC3721087/.

Petrofsky JS, Laymon M, and Lee H (2013) Effect of heat and cold on tendon flexibility and force to flex the human knee. Medical Science Monitor 19 661–670.

Proske U and Gandevia SC (2009) The kinesthetic senses. The Journal of Physiology [Electronic] 58 (17) 4,139–4,146. Available: https://www.ncbi.nlm.nih.gov/pmc/articles/PMC2754351/.

Riemann BL and Lephart SM (2002) The sensorimotor system, part II: The role of proprioception in motor control and functional joint stability. Journal of Athletic Training [Electronic] 37 (1) 80–84. Available: https://www.ncbi.nlm.nih.gov/pmc/articles/PMC164312/.

Riva G (2014) Out of my body: Cognitive neuroscience meets eating disorders. Frontiers in Human Neuroscience 8 236.

Saloman R, Fernandez NB, van Elk M, Vachicouras N, Sabatier F, Tychinskaya A, Llobera J, and Blanke O (2016) Changing motor perception by sensorimotor conflicts and body ownership. Scientific Reports 6 25,847.

Seay JF, Sauer SG, Patel T, and Roy, TC (2016) A history of low back pain affects pelvis and trunk coordination during a sustained manual materials handling task. Journal of Sport and Health Science 5 (1) 52–60.

Simpson MR (2006) Benign joint hyper mobility syndrome: Evaluation, diagnosis, and management. The Journal of the American Osteopathic Association [Electronic] 106 531–536. Available: http://jaoa.org/article.aspx?articleid=2093276.

Stears SS, Fleming R, and Fero LJ (2017) Attenuating physiological arousal through the manipulation of simple hand movements. Applied Psychophysiological Biofeedback 42 (1) 39–50.

Telles S, Gupta TK, Bhardwaj AK, Singh N, Mishra P, Pal DK, and Balkrishna A (2018) Increased mental well-being and reduced state anxiety in teachers after participation in a residential yoga program. Medical Science Monitor Basic Research 24 105–112.

Case study

A client of mine used to have anxiety that would lead to occasional panic attacks. They became frequent enough that her doctor prescribed her anti-anxiety medication to calm her down when she felt one coming on. She didn't love having to take medication, even if it was infrequent. She also had bouts of low back pain that would come on during or directly after periods of high stress.

I taught her alternative nostril breathing, a breathing technique that involves breathing in one nostril and out the other, which she began using on nights when she felt restless. It helped her fall asleep quickly, and she found herself using it when she was feeling stressed.

I also taught her a number of breathing techniques that focus on slowing the breath down. She hasn't had a low back flare-up in a long time, and she generally feels calmer. She did other things, like got stronger, improved her overall proprioception and body awareness, and began a walking program, but the breathing was an important component to improving her mental well-being.

During a recent session, she asked me, "How did you get into the breathing work? It made such a huge difference for me – I no longer have to carry around a bottle of XANAX® to feel calm."

In Chapter 2, I introduced the concept of interoception. Before we dive into breathing and its impact on movement, take a moment to reflect and jot down your impressions of what interoception is and how it relates to awareness.

Interoception is the ability to sense the internal state of the body, such as your breath and heart rate. Researchers haven't quite agreed on an exact definition, but it does seem to be generally agreed that our interoceptive sense is the product of the central nervous system (Ceunen et al. 2016). The somatic nervous system relays information to the brain via peripheral nerve fibers, so you could say the peripheral nervous system chats with the central nervous system, helping you form perceptions about you and the world. (Somatic is defined as relating to the body, so a somatic discipline is one that brings conscious awareness of the body and its functions.)

Interoception is related to a number of things in the academic literature, including:

- pain
- negative emotions
- anxiety
- emotion regulation
- decision making
- subjective time perception
- subjective self-awareness
- food and water intake
- eating disorders
- addiction
- empathy
- meditation

How you perceive and interpret the internal state of the body is closely related to cognition and emotion, which is why when you look at the list above you see things like anxiety, emotion regulation, and decision making. How you interpret the information you are receiving about your internal state contributes to your emotional state or, more simply, how you physically feel affects how you emotionally feel (Garfinkel et al. 2015).

Let's say a student comes in feeling a bit nauseated. The student attributes the nausea to a conversation she is

continued

Case study *continued*

dreading having with her parents and assumes it means the conversation won't go well. If you were to probe a little further, you would find out the egg she ate 3 hours before she arrived tasted kind of funny and is the more probable cause of her nausea. We are constantly making predictions about the world based on past experience and our current reality. The ability to accurately gauge and hone our interoceptive sense gives us an opportunity to make more accurate predictions.

Developing a more accurate interoceptive sense requires practice. (Some scientists consider interoception a sense just like vision, hearing, touch, and, as you learned in the last chapter, proprioception.) All senses can be improved upon with the right input. A Master Sommelier spends years honing their taste and nose so they can accurately depict the flavors and notes on a wine. A student of movement can learn to detect changes in heart and respiration rates, and accurately assess different sensations that arise in the physical body, like whether performing one more round of pull-ups is going to be harmful or injurious to the physical body or whether it's just physically challenging. If it's the latter, performing the extra set once in a while reminds the student they are physically capable of more than they realize, which can build a sense of resilience. Training this form of self-awareness can also create a more balanced relationship with emotions such as anxiety.

I have a client with generalized anxiety disorder. Because she has developed her interoceptive senses, when she feels her heart rate elevating and breath becoming shallower, she acknowledges what she is experiencing in a detached way. This calms her down and enables her to continue functioning, taking her physical symptoms of anxiety down a notch instead of ratcheting them up.

Remember how back in Chapter 1 I said body schema can be affected by a number of factors including physical trauma? The same is true of interoception. Stress, either prolonged or acute, can cause changes in interoception, causing people to become hyperaware or detach completely, correlating with post-traumatic stress disorder (PTSD) and substance use disorders (Price & Hooven 2018).

Joint hypermobility can also lead to a heightened interoceptive sense, anxiety, and heightened perception of pain (Bulbena-Cabre & Bulbena 2018). The more severe forms of joint hypermobility, such as joint hypermobility syndrome and Hypermobile Ehlers-Danlos syndrome (type 3), the greater the correlation to heightened interoception and anxiety (Mallorqui-Bague et al. 2014). We explored the mechanical aspects of joint hypermobility in Chapter 2, but imagine for a moment that your arms don't feel connected to the torso. It's as though if you were to reach for an object just out of reach, your arm would detach from your body. How would that make you feel?

Like you don't really want to reach for anything, right? Now imagine you feel like most of your limbs aren't connected in a cohesive way to the body. Things feel loose and you don't ever quite know where your body parts are located. How would this make you feel? Hyper-vigilant and attentive to your internal signals, perhaps? Worried about injuring yourself? In the very least, there would be a lack of security, as though at any given moment an injury could occur, so the fact that anxiety is correlated to hypermobility shouldn't come as much of a surprise.

The value of variable breathing rates

Breathing can affect both interoception and proprioception. It's unique because it's a physiological function you have partial control over. You can't consciously slow your heart rate down just by focusing on the heart; you can, however, decide you want to breathe slower.

It's also tied to the emotional experience. Things like anxiety and acute stress can cause a shallower breathing pattern. Heightened activation of the sympathetic nervous system (think chronic stress and anxiety) also alters breathing, resulting in shorter inhales and exhales.

Imagine someone silently appeared behind you right now and placed a hand on your shoulder; what would you do? Probably startle and take a quick breath in. The exhale that followed would be short. The shortness of the breath would cause you to breathe more in your chest, which is different from how you breathe when you are relaxed or resting (Harvard Medical School 2015).

A number of things happen during the breath cycle. The breath enters the nose (or mouth), moves into the lungs and fills the lungs with air, changing the pressure inside the thorax. The diaphragm responds by moving down, placing pressure on the organs and moving them down. The pelvic floor responds by moving down. The entire situation reverses on the exhale – the pelvic floor moves up, the diaphragm moves up, the organs shift, the pressure in the lungs decreases as they empty, and the breath moves out. All of this happens with every breath cycle (Novotny & Kravitz 2005).

Breathing also affects heart rate. The inhale speeds the heart up slightly and the exhale slows the heart down slightly. In fact, a healthy heart rate is not one that is metered; "lub–lub–lub" is less optimal than "lub dub … lub dub … lub dub." Another way to think of it is that there is a pause at the end of the inhale and a pause at the end of the exhale, just like there is a pause between heart beats after the heart empties itself of blood and before it refills. It's a lovely, rhythmic system (Russo et al. 2017).

The physiological changes caused by the breath echo throughout the skeleton, causing subtle shifts in position with the inhale and the exhale. The lungs and diaphragm respond to the changes in respiration by changing shape, enlarging and contracting on the inhale and decompressing, getting smaller on the exhale. The ribs shift to accommodate the changes in position and pressure (Bordoni & Zanier 2013).

This can be easily observed by watching a dog dozing on its side. Its belly and ribs rise on the inhale and fall on the exhale. Occasionally, there will be a slightly bigger sigh, causing the belly and ribs to fall a little more obviously.

The breath, like all things in the body, shifts throughout the day depending upon what you're doing. If you are three miles into a moderate six-mile run, the breath will be a little bit quicker than it was right after you ate lunch, corresponding to a faster heart rate. But, assuming the run is something you do regularly, you may barely notice your breathing has changed. It's not uncomfortable in any way, mirroring the sense of comfort and ease you experience while performing this particular activity.

Let's imagine instead that you decide to do wind sprints for the first time in 20 years. By the time you are on your third one, you will feel your breathing becoming uncomfortably shallow and your heart will feel like it's going to leap out of your chest. Why are these two scenarios so different?

The main reason is that the breath corresponds to your perceived exertion, so the harder you feel like you're working, the faster you'll breathe. If you run regularly and are conditioned to running, your perception of work during your six-mile casual run won't be that high. Your breathing will be easier, and you won't feel like you are responding to a potential threat (Zaccaro et al. 2018).

Emotional perceived exertion also causes an increase in respiration rate. Someone who is about to give a lecture to 100 people will likely have a higher respiration rate than someone who is sitting quietly on the couch, reading. The nervous system's perception of moments requiring heightened alertness and attention is situationally dependent, guided by past experiences. The nervous system adjusts to the potential stressor with the appropriate physiological response to meet the demands of the situation and to maximize successful survival.

Anxiety is often accompanied by physiological responses such as an increase in heart rate and breathing. When there is no physiological reason for the increase in heart rate and respiration, that is, there is no lecture to give that requires cortisol to course through the system, or there is nothing physical occurring that requires an increase in metabolic output, the physiological response can feel frightening and result in heightened fear and worry. Exercise, specifically aerobic exercise and resistance training, has been found to be an effective treatment in anxiety-related symptoms. One of the proposed reasons exercise is effective is because it causes similar physiological responses as an anxiety attack. When anxiety-prone individuals see an increase in their ability to cope with the physiological challenges associated with exercise, self-efficacy increases and they feel more able to cope with the physical responses they associate with anxiety (Aylett et al. 2018).

Because breath is both a conscious and an unconscious action, it's possible to teach people how to change their relationship to a situation by changing how they are breathing (Ma et al. 2017). Teaching breath work creates an opportunity for self-awareness, empowering people to slow down, observe, and have control over a basic human function. It also has the added benefit of improving kinesthetic awareness of the structures that support breath, including the abdomen and pelvis.

It's not uncommon for breath work to feel uncomfortable at first, particularly for those with heightened interoceptive sense. Using the proper regressions and drawing awareness to other areas can increase the sense of safety and restore more of a parasympathetic response. We will talk more about safety in Chapter 4, but for now just know that when a person feels safe, it is easier for the person to focus on somatic awareness and, sometimes, focusing on something other than interoceptive awareness is actually a better choice.

The breath is controlled by the autonomic nervous system. This part of the nervous system makes sure all of the functions of being alive are going on in the background, without any conscious thought. Whether you think about inhaling or exhaling, you will inhale and exhale (eventually; even habitual breath-holders breathe occasionally) (Hodges et al. 1997).

The two branches of the autonomic nervous system, the sympathetic nervous system (SNS) and parasympathetic nervous system (PNS) are influenced by how someone breathes (Moore et al. 1998). The inhale is an SNS activity, correlating to the slight increase in heart rate mentioned above. The exhale is a PNS activity, correlating to a slight decrease in heart rate. When the exhale is longer than the inhale, you are spending more time with the PNS activated, which means long exhales can have a calming effect. In fact, slow breathing has been shown to improve feelings of psychological well-being, improve attention, and improve emotional control (Chaudhry & Bhimji 2018; Kiel & Kaiser 2018).

The diaphragm is the muscle that contracts and relaxes when you breathe and is supplied by the phrenic nerve (Neuhuber et al. 2016). When you ask someone to consciously change their breathing patterns by inhaling into different places, slowing the breath down, or breathing through the nose instead of the mouth, the movement of the diaphragm will also be altered. This differs from other physiological functions such as heart rate or digestion. You can't exactly ask someone to fill their heart with blood more slowly, or consciously change how their large intestine is breaking down food. (If you could hack basic physiological functions such as heart function and digestion, you would be worth a lot of money, so please let me know if you figure it out.) Breathing is unique. It isn't something anyone should focus on all of the time, but it can provide valuable feedback about how you are feeling in the moment.

Exercise
Modified alternate nostril breathing

Come into a seated position, with your feet flat on the floor. Observe your breathing, paying attention to how your inhale travels through the body and how the exhale leaves the body. Pay attention to how your jaw feels and your neck. Do those areas feel tight or relaxed? What happens to the jaw and the neck when you inhale? What about when you exhale?

Turn your left palm up towards the ceiling and bring your left thumb and ring finger together a few times.

Now, take the left thumb so that it's barely touching the skin of the left nostril and the left fourth finger so that it's barely touching the skin of the right nostril (Figure 3.1). Apply pressure to the left nostril with the thumb as you inhale, so air only goes in the right nostril. At the top of the inhale, switch, so the left fourth finger is placing enough pressure to close the right nostril and exhale through the left nostril (Figure 3.2). Perform four rounds and then switch hands. Perform four more rounds.

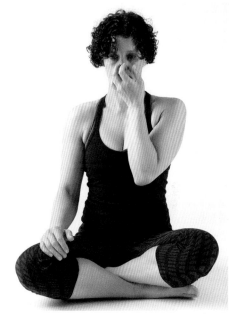

Figure 3.2

After you have finished, rest your hands by your side. Observe your breath. How do you feel? Take your attention to your jaw and neck. Was there any change in the muscle tone of those areas? Remember, the goal isn't to judge. Just notice what you notice.

An effective way to introduce breath work is by giving students something external to focus on. Using the fingers to open and close the nostril in a way that corresponds with the breath focuses attention, which you will learn more about in Chapter 4, and can reduce the panic that is sometimes associated with focused breathing. Focusing on breath can create anxiety, especially if the student has fear around longer exhales, which can initially feel suffocating, like they are going to run out of air. The rhythm of the fingers moving with the breath alters the focus, emphasizing a synchronicity in movement between the fingers and the breathing, down-regulating the SNS.

Breath can also create more motion through the spine. When a person breathes more fully, the ribs move multi-dimensionally. It's like a tube of toothpaste – when you

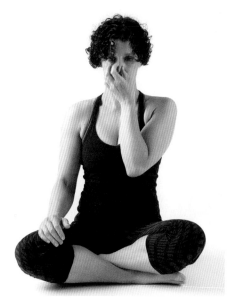

Figure 3.1

inhale and the breath is moving down, your ribs fill in all directions, and your low back fills in all directions. When you exhale, the reverse is true – everything moves toward the center, just like when you squeeze a toothpaste tube. Another way to think of it is inhaling makes the breath move down, taking up space; exhaling makes the breath move up, making the space it was taking up get smaller.

The diaphragm, which is shaped like a lop-sided mushroom and contracts and relaxes every time you inhale and exhale, is mirrored by what is commonly referred to as the pelvic floor, aka the muscles that make up the bowl of the pelvis (Kim & Lee 2013). As a result, breathing that emphasizes the diaphragm can be used as a tool, creating both spinal mobility and spinal stability (Chaitow et al. 2013). Using the breath as a way to improve the connection to spinal movement creates access to movement in a safe, relaxed way; helping people develop less rigidity and more fluidity in their breathing translates into more ease in their day-to-day lives.

When you begin to ask people to notice how their bodies respond to the breath, you are helping them hone interoception and proprioception. Feeling how the ribs move, or feeling the sensation of work in the abdominals during certain breathing exercises, strengthens the mind–body connection and creates a more complete body schema through better body awareness.

Exercise
Prone breathing in spinal flexion

Come on to your hands and knees. Drop your hips to your heels and let your spine round. Place your crossed palms under your forehead or along the sides of your body with your palms towards the ceiling and your forehead on the floor (Figure 3.3).

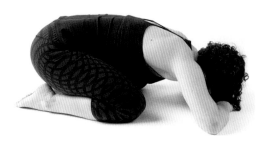

Figure 3.3

Imagine two hands on your back, right between your shoulder blades. As you inhale through your nose, see if you can make the area under the imaginary hands broaden with your breath. As you exhale, "sigh" out of your mouth and allow the area between the shoulder blades to soften. Feel your ribs moving in, making your mid-back smaller. As you inhale, feel the area broaden. Repeat for four to six breath cycles. (If the initial position feels too intense, use pillows to support your thighs against your knees and/or your head.)

Breathing into the mid-back and emphasizing the rib expansion and contraction enables students to feel a connection between the breath and how it affects the rib cage region. The cue "ribs down and in," while well intentioned, is often misinterpreted when students don't understand how the ribs move. Teaching students to feel rib movement makes it easier to translate cueing of the ribs in different positions.

At a workshop I was teaching, Anna shared that she used to always feel a sensation of tightness in her mid-back area, but after the last workshop I had taught, the tightness disappeared, never to return. She correlated a specific breathing exercise to the disappearance of her mid-back tightness. Why did breathing make a difference?

Think about the ribs for a minute. How are they oriented? The first 10 ribs connect the sternum (aka the breast bone) to the vertebrae on the back. The lower two ribs "float," which means they originate on the last two thoracic vertebrae and don't attach anywhere on the front.

I mentioned earlier that one of the things the breath does is move the ribs. Anna was a habitual chest breather, which means her breath made her chest rise and fall, but her ribs didn't move laterally or posteriorly when she inhaled (to the side or to the back). Her ribs weren't getting used, so the muscles that supported the ribs weren't getting used. They felt tight because they weren't changing position.

A term that is commonly used when discussing breath work is "diaphragmatic breathing," but what, exactly, does that mean? Maybe you've asked people to belly breathe or instructed people to "breathe like a baby," but is that actually diaphragmatic breathing? (And do many people actually know how babies breathe?)

A common mistake people make when they are teaching diaphragmatic breathing is that they ask people to breathe just into their belly. The problem with this is the belly moves because the organs move down, because the diaphragm moves down, and because the lungs fill. The belly moving is one link in a chain of events: a result of what happens above it, not a cause.

As things shift during the inhale, if the breath is efficient, the low back, the ribs, the chest, and the pelvic floor all move as well. Breathing is a 360° movement, not just a front–back movement. The next series of exercises are designed to improve awareness of how you breathe and teach different focal points for the inhale and exhale.

Practical application

I was filming a segment for an online low back awareness course. The person I was using as a demo for the breathing portion was someone I hadn't trained before, and when he agreed to do it, we didn't discuss anything other than his low back health.

At the end of the breathing work, he mentioned his shoulder felt more mobile. One of the breathing exercises we did emphasized breathing across the chest and getting expansion using air in the area near his arm pit. By getting a little bit of movement in his upper ribs and across his collarbone, his arm felt like it had more room to move.

This is because breathing can affect more than just the diaphragm. It influences how well your shoulder moves, your experience of mobility in your hips, and how you use the muscles around your torso. Spending a little bit of time paying attention to your breathing and gaining control over how you breathe can make your body feel more free and your mind feel more calm.

How to use the breathing exercises

Breathing exercises can be used as a restorative practice to down-regulate the nervous system. They can also be used as a pre-cursor to abdominal work (particularly if the person struggles with breath holding or uses bracing strategies such as doming the abdominal wall or bearing down the abdominals to stabilize), or as a way to cool-down and reset after a challenging workout. I often give breathing exercises as homework to new clients. Because they feel gentle and don't require any equipment (they can often be done in bed), adherence is usually high. This begins to develop a habit of awareness and movement done at home, away from a studio setting, and eventually (it is hoped) leading to more movement.

Exercise
Breathing observation

Lie on your back, with your knees bent and your feet flat. Observe your breath, like you did earlier, noticing which parts of your body fill when you inhale and which parts of your body get heavier when you exhale. Do this for four breaths.

Shift your awareness to breathing in through your nose for a count of four and exhale out through your nose or mouth for a count of four. Do this for four breaths.

Now, breathe in through your nose for a count of four. Exhale out through your nose or mouth for a count of six. Do this for four breaths.

Finally, inhale through your nose for a count of four and exhale out through your nose or mouth for a count of eight.

Take a moment to observe your breathing without counting the lengths of the breath. Does it feel any different?

Why long exhales?

When you ask people to take an exhale that is longer than they are used to, they may feel like they don't have enough air to exhale for that long. The lungs always have air in them that never makes it to the circulatory system, commonly referred to as dead space (Intagliata et al. 2019). The dead space can be thought of as extra air, which means people often have more air than they think they do. If a person's habit is to take short exhales, the nervous system will say, "Hey, wait a minute. This is different. I don't know if this is safe. I need to inhale NOW." The strong panicky feeling that arises, causing people to feel like they need to inhale, is perfectly normal. Like all things, learning to pause at the end of an exhale can be improved with practice.

Dead space is reduced during slow breathing because ventilatory efficiency improves, so teaching people how to exhale longer isn't just safe, it makes the respiratory system more efficient. It's like minimalism – why keep old air around that you aren't using?

If you notice someone feels anxious when attempting longer exhales, see how long they can exhale without feeling panicky. With practice, they will feel safer exhaling longer, and eventually may even begin to feel a sense of calm or relaxation.

Exercise
Breathing across the chest into the finger tips

Lie on your back, with your knees bent and your feet flat on the floor. Reach your right arm out so it makes a "T" with your body. Place your left fingertips on the collar bone where it meets the breast bone.

As you inhale through your nose, move your left fingers out across the collar bone to where it meets the shoulder, gently stroking the area.

Exhale; trace the fingers in the opposite direction to where the collar bone meets the breast bone. Breathe slowly and see if you can move your fingers at the same rate as your breath. Perform four breaths and switch sides.

After you have performed four breaths on the other side, stay on your back with your arms in a "T." Feel your breath expand under your collar bones to your shoulders when you inhale. Feel how that area relaxes and softens on the exhale. Perform four breaths.

Take a moment to observe your breath. How does it feel?

When you ask someone to focus on the breath across the chest and under the collar bones, you direct their attention to the expansion and contraction of the lungs with the breath. The lungs are interesting from an anatomical perspective, with three lobes on the right and two on the left. The bottom of the lungs lies in front of the T5, T6, T7 vertebrae (basically, the middle thoracic spine). The lungs change shape during the inhale and get bigger; on the exhale, they get smaller. They function to transfer oxygen from the air to the blood, which they do via a specialized cell membrane called alveoli (Powers & Dhamoon 2019).

The collar bones are designed to move when the breast bone moves and when the shoulders move. Movement at the sternoclavicular joint (the meeting place of the breast bone and sternum), occurs to allow transmission of force from the shoulder blade and the arm (Kiel & Kaiser 2019).

The sternum keeps the organs safe and is an attachment point for the cartilage from the first seven ribs (Safarini & Bordoni 2019). When you inhale and exhale, the cartilage of the sternum allows the sternum to move with the breath, just like the ribs move with the breath. Another way of looking at this is the breath causes a little wave of responses throughout the bones of the upper extremities.

Placing the fingers on the collar bone and tracing the collar bone with the breath does two things: it creates a clearer image in the body schema of where the collar bone is, improving kinesthesia. Tracing the collar bone with the inhale and the exhale also increases interoception by drawing attention to the breath.

Exercise
Allowing the ribs to move

Lie on your back with your knees bent and your feet flat. Begin with your arms and hands in a comfortable position and place your attention on the mid-back. Does it make contact with the floor? As you breathe, do you feel any movement through the mid-back? If you are unclear where the mid-back is located, it's the part of your spine right under your shoulder blades; the low back begins right below the last rib.

Place your hands on your lower ribs (Figure 3.4). Begin breathing in through your nose and out through your mouth, like you are quietly sighing. As you exhale, use your hands to gently guide your ribs toward the floor and toward the pelvis, so they are moving down and in. As you inhale, see if you can feel the ribs expand without lifting up toward the ceiling. Stay here for four breaths.

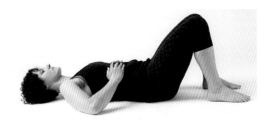

Figure 3.4

Now, come into a seated position with your mid-back against a wall or against a straight-backed chair, whichever is most comfortable for you. Rest your hands on your thighs. As you inhale, see if you can feel the back of the ribs lightly pressing into the surface behind you. Exhale, maintain the rib contact, but notice what happens to the ribs in the front of the body. Can you feel them moving down? Stay here for four breaths.

Lie on your back one more time, with your knees bent and your feet flat on the floor. Take a moment to observe your next four breaths. Where do you feel movement when you inhale? What about when you exhale?

Exercise
Breathing into the pelvis

Lie down on your stomach, with your forehead on the floor and your arms in a diamond shape around your head. If you are uncomfortable with your arms overhead, place them by your sides or place them under your forehead.

Imagine your breath is like an elevator moving from the top floor (the nose) to the bottom floor (the pelvic floor). Inhale; follow the breath down until you feel movement in your pelvis. You might feel the front of the pelvis pressing a little more into the floor. As you exhale, trace the elevator back up until it exits out of the nose. Perform eight breaths. You may begin to feel your low back widening and the pelvis moving subtly as you breathe.

Chapter 3

Turn over on to your back so your knees are bent and your feet are flat on the floor. Take eight more slow breaths. Can you feel the breath moving down as you inhale? Is your low back in contact with the floor? Don't force anything; just observe.

During quiet inhalation, the diaphragm contracts and moves down. The pelvic floor also relaxes and moves down, mirroring the movement of the diaphragm. During quiet exhalation, the diaphragm recoils passively, moving up; the pelvic floor responds by contracting and moving up (Kim & Lee 2013). (Note, the diaphragm moves up by relaxing while the pelvic floor moves up by contracting. We will discuss the contraction and relaxation of the pelvic floor in more detail in Chapter 9.) Paying attention to how the body responds during breath can improve general body awareness in both the pelvis and low back in addition to the ribs, sternum, and shoulders. (Who knew breathing was such a total body activity?) Becoming more connected to the different places breath can be directed continues to improve a person's accuracy of their body schema, improving both integration of body parts into movement and overall awareness.

There are a number of muscles that attach the ribs to your pelvis. Often, when people think about the "core" muscles, they think about the rectus abdominis, the six-pack muscle on the front of the abdomen that's visible on a well-muscled individual. Underneath the rectus abdominis are a number of muscles that create intra-abdominal pressure and support the spine. The transversus abdominis, a belt-like muscle that runs horizontally along the front of the torso, actually connects to the diaphragm at the ribs, allowing both muscles to create stability throughout the spine and trunk. The diaphragm, of course, is the breathing muscle, so it would stand to reason breathing can lead to the sensation of work in the abdominal musculature, especially if someone isn't used to letting the ribs move with the breath. The sensation of work could also be thought of as force acting on the musculoskeletal system. I noted earlier that force is a way to improve proprioception, so feeling the abdominals during the breathing exercises improves proprioception as well.

Exercise
Breathing with the arms

Come into a comfortable standing position with your arms by your sides. As you inhale, imagine the breath moving all of the way across the collarbones to the fingertips. As you exhale, feel how the breath moves out, across the collarbones and out of the nose. It's the same sensation you worked on in the exercise "breathing across the chest into the fingertips." Allow your arms to respond to the breath, which just means that if they want to move a little bit on the inhale, let them move, and if they want to shift on the exhale, let them shift. Stay here for four breaths.

Now, take your arms up as though they were loosely holding a large ball in front of your chest. As you inhale, let the breath move your fingertips away from one another. As you exhale, let your fingertips come toward one another. Let your arms move at the same rate as your breath, so it's as though the breath is moving the arms. Perform for six breath cycles.

Lie down on your back with your knees bent and your feet flat. Your arms will make a "T" with the body. Inhale through the nose and exhale through the nose. Can you feel the breath moving across the chest toward the fingertips?

Remember that one of the things that provides feedback to the brain about the body's location in space is the receptors in the skin that detect touch. One of the reasons standing exercises often feel more challenging than supine exercises for people to "get right" is because there is no longer pressure from the floor along the length of the body, providing sensory feedback to the brain. By alternating a standing position with a supine position, you give your students or clients an opportunity to check the accuracy of their perceptions, assisting with the learning process.

The arms, of course, aren't actually breathing, but tuning in to the breath activates the PNS, reducing the feeling of tension through the arms, neck, and upper back.

The arms begin to feel light and respond to the subtle changes that occur with the breath, creating an integrated movement.

Exercise
Breathing into the leg

Come into a tall kneeling position as though you were standing on your knees. Take a moment to place your fingers on your two front hip bones, the knobby points in the front of your pelvis where pants often sit.

Move the front hip bones up toward your ribs and then move them down away from your ribs. Make the motion small, focusing on the subtle movement in the pelvis. Do this six to eight times.

Find a position in your pelvis that feels balanced and place your hands gently on the tops of the thighs and inhale through your nose. Imagine the elevator moving all of the way down to the pelvis. You may feel the hip bones move up slightly, or the pressure against your hands change. As you exhale slowly, feel the breath move up and out. You may feel the hip bones move down slightly or the pressure against your hands lessening.

Continue breathing, and see if you can feel the effects of the breath moving all of the way down the legs as you inhale. As you exhale, feel how the legs and pelvis respond to the exhale. Perform for four breaths.

Lie down on your back, with your knees bent and your feet flat. Rest your hands in a comfortable position, and feel what parts of yourself respond to the inhale and to the exhale for the next four breaths.

The femur connects to the pelvis via the acetabulofemoral joint. Movement is created by either the femur moving around the pelvis or the pelvis moving around the femur. Creating subtle movement with the breath fine tunes the kinesthetic sense of the hip socket and the different ways movement can occur. (We will discuss this in more detail in Chapter 9.)

Exercise
Hissing breath

Lie down on your back, with your knees bent and your feet flat. Rest your hands in a comfortable position.

Inhale gently through the nose. As you exhale, make a "sss" sound, as though you were hissing. Exhale as long as you can and feel what happens in your ribs as you exhale. When you get to the bottom of the exhale, pause for a moment with the tongue on the roof of the mouth before you inhale softly and slowly through your nose. Repeat for four to six breaths.

Remain on your back. Let your eyes close, and feel the weight of your body against the floor as you take four to six more slow, easy breaths.

I mentioned that long exhales are challenging because they can cause feelings of anxiety and concern that there isn't enough air. Creating a task-based exhale, such as making a hissing sound, naturally slows the exhale without overly focusing on it. This allows you to introduce long exhales in a way that feels safe for the individual. Certain sounds, like the "s" sound, the "f" sound, and the "ch" sound, naturally slow down the exhale and may cause the sensation of abdominal work or coughing, re-enforcing kinesthetic awareness and improving proprioception. When you teach slow exhales, it's important to make sure people are doing it easily, not forcing the breath or bearing down, allowing the student to maximize the relaxation benefits associated with down-regulating the PNS.

You probably noticed that all of the exercises end with the student on their back, actively observing what they are feeling. This gives them an opportunity to feel their body against the floor. It also creates an opportunity for the student to recognize when things have changed, which is valuable if your goal is to instill a growth mindset: feeling change happen in a short time span reinforces the fact that students are capable of learning and changing.

This isn't the only way, of course, and these exercises aren't the only ways to teach breathing. One of the best aspects about teaching movement is that once you understand the concepts, you can use your creativity to develop exercises that utilize the ideas and enhance what you are trying to teach. Not every exercise will work for every person; the more options you have via positions and cueing, the better the chance you will be able to find a variation that works for the person in front of you.

It's important to remember the body is incredibly adaptable. Tissues change and become stronger and more flexible with the right stimulus, supporting the physical structure during physical activity and daily life. The neuromuscular system is the same way. It's adaptable and learns with repeated exposure, constantly figuring out how to be more efficient with the information it's given. When you take the time to teach the subtleties of something like the breath, you are potentially creating opportunities for better interoceptive awareness. You are offering people a chance to find a little more ease physically and emotionally.

Practical application

Before you move on to the next chapter, set a timer for 5 minutes. Spend the next 5 minutes experimenting with ways to breathe in different positions, observing how breath subtly affects the rest of the physical structure. If you find something you like or find interesting, take a moment to write it down or film it so you can return to it again. (I have lost many great exercises I "invented" because I didn't take the time to make a note of them. The extra minute it takes to note the exercise is well worth it.)

References

Aylett E, Small N, and Bower P (2018) Exercise in the treatment of clinical anxiety in general practice – a systematic review and meta-analysis. BMC Health Service Research 18 (1) 559.

Bordoni B and Zanier E (2013) Anatomic connections of the diaphragm: Influence of respiration on the body system. Journal of Multidisciplinary Healthcare [Electronic] 6 281–291. Available: https://www.ncbi.nlm.nih.gov/pmc/articles/PMC3731110/.

Bulbena-Cabre A and Bulbena A (2018) Anxiety and joint hypermobility: An unexpected association. Current Psychiatry 14 (4) 15–21.

Ceunen E, Vlaeyen JWS, and Van Diest I (2016) On the origins of interoception. Frontiers in Psychology 7 743.

Chaitow L, Gilbert C, and Bradley D (2013) Recognizing and treating breathing disorders, 2nd edn. London: Churchill Livingston.

Chaudhry R and Bhimji SS (2018) Anatomy, thorax, lungs. Treasure Island, FL: StatPearls Publishing. Available: https://www.ncbi.nlm.nih.gov/books/NBK470197/.

Garfinkel SN, Seth AK, Barrett AB, Suzuki K, and Critchley HD (2015) Knowing your own heart: Distinguishing interoceptive accuracy from interoceptive awareness. Biological Psychology 104 65–74.

Harvard Medical School (2015) Relaxation techniques: Breath control helps quell errant stress response. Boston, MA: Harvard Health Publishing. Available: https://www.health.harvard.edu/mind-and-mood/relaxation-techniques-breath-control-helps-quell-errant-stress-response.

Hodges PW, Butler JE, McKenzie DK, and Gandevia SC (1997) Contraction of the human diaphragm during rapid postural adjustments. Journal of Physiology [Online] 505 (2) 539–548. Available: https://www.ncbi.nlm.nih.gov/pmc/articles/PMC1160083/.

Intagliata S, Rizzo A, and Gossman WG (2019) Physiology, lung dead space. Treasure Island, FL: StatPearls Publishing.

Kiel J and Kaiser K (2018) Sternoclavicular joint injury. Treasure Island, FL: StatPearls Publishing. Available: https://www.ncbi.nlm.nih.gov/books/NBK507894/.

Kiel J and Kaiser K (2019) Sternoclavicular joint injury. Treasure Island, FL: StatPearls Publishing.

Kim E and Lee H (2013) The effects of deep abdominal muscle strengthening exercises on respiratory function and lumbar stability. Journal of Physical Therapy Science [Electronic] 25 (6) 663–665. Available: https://www.ncbi.nlm.nih.gov/pmc/articles/PMC3805012/.

Ma X, Yue ZQ, Gong Z-Q, Zhang H, Duan N-Y, Shi Y-T, Wei G-X, and Li Y-F (2017) The effect of diaphragmatic breathing on attention, negative affect and stress in healthy adults. Frontiers in Psychology [Electronic] 8 874. Available: https://www.ncbi.nlm.nih.gov/pmc/articles/PMC5455070/.

Mallorqui-Bague, Garfinkel SN, Engels M, Eccles JA, Pailhez G, Bulbena A, and Critchley HD (2014) Neuroimaging and psychophysiological investigation of the link between anxiety, enhanced affective reactivity and interception in people with joint hypermobility. Frontiers in Psychology 5 1,162.

Moore KL, Agur AMR, and Dalley AF II (1998) Essential clinical anatomy. Philadelphia, PA: Wolters Kluwer Health.

Neuhuber W, Lyer S, Alexiou C, and Buder T (2016) Anatomy and blood supply of the sternum, in Horch R, Willy C, and Kutschka I (eds) Deep sternal wound infections. Berlin, Heidelberg: Springer.

Novotny S and Kravitz L (2005) The science of breathing. Albuquerque: University of New Mexico. Available: https://www.unm.edu/~lkravitz/Article%20folder/Breathing.html

Powers KA and Dhamoon AS (2019) Physiology, pulmonary, ventilation and perfusion. Treasure Island, FL: StatPearls Publishing.

Price CJ and Hooven C (2018) Interoceptive awareness skills for emotion regulation: Theory and approach of mindful awareness in body-oriented therapy (MABT). Frontiers in Psychology 9 798.

Russo MA, Santarelli DM, and O'Rourke D (2017) The physiological effects of slow breathing in the healthy human. Breathe [Electronic] 13 (4) 298–309. Available: https://www.ncbi.nlm.nih.gov/pmc/articles/PMC5709795/.

Safarini OA and Bordoni B (2019) Aanatomy, thorax, ribs. Treasure Island, FL: StatPearls Publishing.

Zaccaro A, Piarulli A, Laurino M, Garbella E, Menicucci D, Neri B, and Gemignani A (2018) How breath-control can change your life: A systematic review on psycho-physiological correlates of slow breathing. Frontiers in Human Neuroscience [Electronic] 12 353. Available: https://www.ncbi.nlm.nih.gov/pmc/articles/PMC6137615/.

Case study

I have a client who has a lot of stress in his life and a fair amount of discomfort in the right side of the body. He has had low back pain on the right side, and his right hand swells occasionally. He has had it imaged, and there is no structural reason for the swelling, but still it shows up once in a while.

I recently noticed while he was doing a single arm mobility exercise that when his right hand reaches up for a bar, his torso moves to the right. When his left hand moves up, his torso stays in the center.

The technical word for this is differentiation. On the left-hand side, he is able to differentiate (or separate) arm movement from torso movement. On the right-hand side, the movements are coupled, so they happen together.

He couldn't feel his torso shifting when he reached the right arm up, so I showed him what it looked like on me, both what happened on his right side and on his left. As I finished my demonstration and looked at him, I could tell it was like a lightbulb going off. "I notice I drift to the right in the car. I just never really considered that it was a problem. It feels like work to stay more in the center." We discussed strategies for driving, and over the course of the next several sessions, I worked on creating awareness through the right torso and arm so he could feel when his torso moved to the right, and introduced ways to lift the arm without the torso shifting.

This particular client has a good handle on using words to describe what's happening in his body. The word "drift" is a perfect description of his habit to slowly make his way to the right side of his body. While he couldn't feel it happening when he was standing, understanding the sensation when he was seated made it easier to eventually cultivate the same body awareness in other positions. You can't change what you can't feel, and perhaps you can't feel what you can't articulate.

(Update: Not only does he no longer shift his torso to the right when he raises his right arm, his back in general is feeling much better. Changing a daily habit, that is, the way he sat in the car, made a dramatic difference in the way he used his body.)

During the breathing exercises in the last chapter, I drew attention to the ribs, chest, mid-back, and pelvis, creating a focal point to decrease mind wandering.

There were also observation cues, directed toward observing the present experience in a way that was non-critical or judgmental. These types of cues also place the practitioner in the present moment.

Both of these are meditation techniques called focused attention and open monitoring, respectively. Focused attention is required to learn a new skill or when you are working on something challenging (Wulf 2007). It's probably obvious, but when attention is split, it's more difficult to do a new or challenging task well (Yeung & Monsell 2003).

It's important to notice the emphasis on new or challenging tasks. Performing a task that's automatic, that is, where you don't have to focus on it, like walking, gives the brain an opportunity to make connections and actually boosts creativity (Oppezzo & Schwartz 2014). The goal isn't to ask people to focus all of the time, but to create opportunities where focusing is required. The contrast between focus and mind wandering becomes more impactful, and the ability to focus becomes easier when students have an opportunity to practice it regularly.

Learning implies that there is a challenge of some sort. If you already know the information or how to accomplish a specific task, you wouldn't need to obtain it – you would already have the necessary mental or neuromuscular knowledge to be successful. The breathing exercises, for example, give students a chance to feel their breathing

continued

43

habits and teach them other ways to breathe. That's all any exercise of movement is, really: an opportunity to learn how to do something new or in a different way.

There is a model called the Challenge Point Framework that suggests the best way to learn a motor skill is for the learner to be actively involved in problem solving to find movement solutions (Pollack et al. 2014). Think of it this way: I could ask you to take a big step out to the side by bending and externally rotating your right knee, while keeping your torso upright, or I could set up an obstacle on the right side of your body and ask you to step over it without hitting the obstacle. Which scenario is more interesting and more engaging? Probably the second one, right? Interacting with the environment creates context, and context is generally more meaningful for learning than performing a movement without context.

A number of tasks outside of exercise and movement require focused attention, such as learning to play a musical instrument, putting together a puzzle, or writing a book. Applying focused attention taps into the mindful part of movement and makes it easier to apply concepts related to learning in the movement setting.

What if you are teaching someone a skill they have been practicing for years? How can you make a task that has become mindless more mindful?

One possible answer is to introduce novelty and ask the student to perform the task in a new way. You can do this through directed cueing (cueing the head action in a squat, for instance, instead of the feet, is unusual and will change the experience of the student). You can also ask the person to perform an externally based task that requires the movement. If we stay with the squat example, you could ask someone to play catch with someone else while squatting. It's impossible to check Instagram while trying to catch

a ball and squat at the same time. (Or maybe it's not. But I don't recommend trying it.)

Another illustration of this in your everyday life is the way you brush your teeth. Which hand do you usually use to brush? Do you brush up and down or side to side? What happens if you switch the hand you use to brush? How does that feel? It immediately requires more focus and attention, right? You can't do it on autopilot like you normally do. You have made something familiar and rote new again.

This isn't to say that you should ask people to change every activity they do. That would be exhausting and a huge waste of energy – habits and routines are developed so people can get through the day easily and have energy for things that require a lot of attention. However, piquing people's curiosity about how they do things, like carry groceries, reach for a glass, or get up from a chair, can inspire curiosity, develop kinesthetic awareness, and create a clearer body image. Plus, it makes the body and how it's used interesting. When you ask people, "Can you do this another way?" they are forced to pause, consider their normal strategy, and reflect on what other options they may have available.

Let's return to the squat example. People are generally cued to squat a specific way, depending on context. In a yoga class, maybe they are asked to externally rotate the feet, lower the hips down to the heels, rest for a few breaths, and then return to a standing position. In a gym setting, maybe it's with an external load, feet strongly pushing into the floor, knees externally rotated.

What happens if you ask people to squat with their feet staggered? Or with one foot angled in and one foot angled out? Or with one foot lifted? Or at varied depth? Or leading with their sitting bones (or initiating from their knees or their eyes)?

Exercise
Squatting multiple ways

Set a timer for 2 minutes.

Squat in as many different ways you can think of over the course of the next 2 minutes. Vary feet, depth, arms, tempo, and any other variable you can think of.

When the timer goes off, spend a moment reflecting. What felt familiar? What felt like a challenge?

Research suggests when you introduce variability during practice, motor skill learning happens faster and motor schema formation is improved. Motor schema can be thought of as the moving body schema. Neuroscientists speculate the brain holds a constantly updated status of the body shape and posture that's determined by the (mostly) unconscious integration of proprioceptive signals. This image is a more conscious, or readily accessible, representation of the body (Chua et al. 2019; Morasso et al. 2015). Asking students to perform a skill like squatting in a variety of ways will not only make them better squatters, it will also make them more conscious of their body and how it moves.

Focused attention gives students an opportunity to practice a technique often used in meditation without lying down on their backs and actually meditating. Focused-attention meditation may improve cognitive control, which is the process the brain uses to determine how goals or plans influence a person's behavior (Chan et al. 2018). Cognitive control is supported by goal-directed thoughts and flexible, adaptive responses, which is exactly what you are teaching someone when you ask them to squat different ways or squat while catching a ball. Focused attention is like any skill. The more you ask someone to practice it, the easier it becomes, and the easier it is to find a balance between mindlessness and mindfulness. (Again, habits and routines are good! And so is paying attention once in a while.)

Case study

A woman was referred to me because she had chronic low back pain. She was hoping to improve her relationship to movement, gain confidence, and avoid injury.

The first time I met her, I noticed she had a tendency to hyperextend her knees (she is naturally very flexible) and stand with her right leg back. She did it every time she was standing; it quickly became obvious her standing position was so habitual, she didn't realize she was doing it.

I brought it to her attention, and asked her to pay attention to how she stood between our sessions. She came in two weeks later and said she was surprised how often she caught herself standing with her knees hyperextended.

It's been two years; her back pain is much better, and she no longer habitually stands with her knees hyperextended or her right leg always back. She has other options for standing. She also no longer has to think about how she stands. She naturally gravitates toward positions that allow her to stand for long periods without discomfort.

Chapter 4

Habits and pain

If introducing variability into regular movement patterns enhances mindfulness/focused attention, improves cognitive control, and improves motor schema, what happens when people aren't exposed to moving in a variable way? What if people move in a way that is predictable?

I touched on this earlier when I mentioned our bodies and our minds evolved to adapt to a variety of surfaces and movement puzzles. "Look! There is a tree in the middle of my path. How shall I get over it?" isn't a question most people find themselves asking on a regular basis in today's world.

This lack of variability can lead to movements that become habitual. Think of habitual movement as movement that is done in a very similar way, adapting to the needs of the situation. For instance, pretend John the accountant doesn't have many opportunities during his daily life to reach his arms overhead. The actions that accompany shoulder flexion, such as scapular upward rotation, will be "forgotten" and not integrated into John's motor schema as an option for shoulder blade movement. Over time, John may adopt a strategy of elevating the shoulder to lift the arm, bypassing scapular upward rotation. Because he isn't asked to lift his arm very often, this strategy has been working just fine, but lately he has noticed his neck feels stiff and there is a general sensation of tightness through his mid-back.

Now, imagine John is invited to a yoga class. He attends, because he's always been curious about yoga and the potential health benefits. The class of the day is a level I vinyasa class with an emphasis on warrior II. Partway through the class, John is experiencing significant neck tension and discomfort. The yoga teacher begins to instruct the students to imagine their arms are light, fully supported by the structure of their shoulder blades and collar bones. John is confused, because he doesn't understand how to move the shoulder blades or what the collar bones have to do with anything, but intrigued, because it sounds like the yoga teacher is talking about something that might be helpful if he could only figure out what the teacher means.

John has a habit of lifting his arms in a way that, while not efficient, works for him. The "new" movement of warrior II performed repeatedly highlights his habitual strategy; the teacher's cueing lets John know he might be able to perform the movement in a different way; in the meantime, he begins to pay attention to how he currently lifts his arms.

Researchers Susana Ramirez-Vizcaya and Tom Froese suggest that habits aren't rigid structures. While they may be performed in a way that appears thoughtless or automatic, they are plastic, capable of changing and adapting to the body and the environment (Ramirez-Vizcaya & Froese 2019).

One of the many aspects of habit formation is environmental context. If someone walks past the pantry on their way to the study, perhaps a habit forms where every time they walk to the study, they open the pantry and grab a handful of almonds. If they were to move into a different house where they didn't walk past the pantry when they walked to the study, there is a high likelihood the habit of eating a handful of almonds would disappear. Because habits are activated by recurring environmental cues, changing the environment can be instrumental in changing the habit (Wood & Runger 2016). John-the-new-yoga-student is not only in a new environment (the yoga studio), he is also being asked to focus on how he lifts his shoulder, a perfect context for learning.

I mentioned earlier that posture does not necessarily correlate with pain; neither does a specific movement habit. But movement habits can contribute to inefficiency and lack of coordination and, if there is pain present, it's worthwhile to see if introducing movement variability decreases the sensation of discomfort.

Case study

Jane lives part-time on the Monterey Peninsula. Every year when she arrives for our first visit, I ask her how she's feeling and she gives me a quick and thorough report.

A couple of years ago on her first visit back, she said she had been experiencing discomfort in her right shoulder. She had mentioned it to the doctor and he had run a series of standard muscular tests to make sure she didn't have a rotator cuff tear. She didn't, but she still had discomfort.

I had her reach for an object and noticed there was no movement in her shoulder blade. When you reach far enough forward, the shoulder blade moves forward. It's almost like the shoulder blade is an extension of the arm. Her habit had become to just reach with the humerus. Her afferent nervous system had become sensitized to the strategy, causing her shoulder to ache when she reached.

I taught her how to reach with the entire arm, allowing the shoulder blade to protract when she had something in front of her. I also had her work on reaching at different angles, so that she could feel how many ways the shoulder blade moved.

After four weeks of regularly warming up with reaching exercises, I asked her how her shoulder was doing. "Fine," she said. "You cured me." All I did was help her pay attention to how she used her arm daily, giving her more options.

Another way to look at habit is as a process where a stimulus generates an impulse to act (Luque 2017). The impulse to act becomes so routine, you don't think about it. With regards to your movement habits, unless you see yourself in a video or someone points your tendencies out to you, they can be difficult to feel. Paying attention is a great substitute for videoing or coaching, and a little bit of mindfulness can go a long way.

Changing habits takes time and, as I mentioned earlier, many of our habits exist to make our lives easier. It's when habits become so strong you forget that there are any other options that they become a problem.

The stages of motor learning

I mentioned above that focused attention is required to learn a new task. It is believed that sensorimotor learning, or learning that requires an element of motor control, happens in three distinct phases: the cognitive stage, the associative stage, and the autonomous stage (Taylor & Ivry 2015).

The cognitive stage is the introduction to a task. The student is introduced to clearly defined movement goals and asked to figure out the appropriate sequence of actions required to accomplish the task. This can also be thought of as the coordination phase, where basic skill coordination is attained for successful completion of the movement. Focused attention is required during the cognitive phase while the student struggles with basic task completion.

Once basic coordination is attained and the movement no longer feels awkward, the student moves into the associative phase. The student is now able to successfully complete the basic elements of the task, but is still working on smoothing out specific elements of the movement. Attention is focused on details that will make the movement more coordinated or improve the student's ability to complete the task successfully. This phase still requires focused attention, but it's easier for the student to know where to place their attention (in the cognitive stage, it can feel like there are so many things to think about, it's difficult to know which aspect of the movement should be the primary point of focus).

Finally, there's the autonomous stage. The movement no longer needs to be thought about – it can be executed in an almost automatic fashion, but learning still occurs as the student figures out how to adapt to a variety of environments and consistently execute the skill.

Remember John, the new yoga student from earlier in the chapter who was intrigued by the idea that he could lift his arms differently, but wasn't sure how to do it? Warrior II is a yoga pose that requires a straight back leg, a bent front knee, specific torso placement, and, depending on whose class you're in, specific foot alignment. This is before you even get to the arm position. Already, there are a lot of things to think about. It's no wonder John couldn't discern how to lift the arms differently. What would have made him more successful at learning how to lift his arms in this position?

If he were introduced to different strategies for lifting the arm in a position that felt more secure and more comfortable, he would have been able to focus on just moving the arms. Whenever someone is placed in a position that feels foreign, the neuromuscular system has to assess the safety of the position, figure out the strategies available to accomplish the position, and then figure out how much muscular activation is needed to maintain the position. This is a form of stress, and though being exposed to a new position is generally good stress (or eustress), it's still going to feel like a challenge. Had John been sitting on a stool or bolster, or even lying down, the concept of lifting the arm in a variety of ways would have been more successful because he had less to focus on. Because lifting the arm is a fairly basic movement, John would move through the stages of learning quickly, enabling him to then be able to execute warrior II more efficiently.

This doesn't mean John will have the muscular strength or endurance to hold the pose for long periods of time.

Getting stronger takes time (usually about 8 weeks, depending on a variety of factors, including repeated exposure to the specific task), so while John may understand how to move the arms in a more efficient way, it doesn't mean he won't experience muscular effort (Sbardelotto et al. 2019). Thinking about his arms, however, will be one less thing he needs to do while trying to figure out the more complex mechanics of warrior II.

Neuroception

If the goal is to maximize learning, reducing the sensation of threat is important. Neuroception is a term that was introduced by researcher Stephen Porges (2009) to describe the process of determining whether environmental and visceral features are safe, dangerous, or life-threatening. In the same way that kinesthetic awareness is different from proprioception, neuroception differs from cognitive perception because it occurs subconsciously, underneath the surface of conscious thought and awareness. When neuroception deems an environment safe, SNS activity is dampened, creating an optimal environment for focused attention and learning.

This doesn't mean you can't learn or perform in a situation that feels unsafe. High-level athletes are asked to perform in stressful situations all of the time. Yuri Hanin (2000: 65) coined the term "individual zones of optimal functioning" (IZOF) to describe the optimal emotional state necessary to perform well. Heightened SNS response is necessary for performance (if you are ready to take a nap, chances are high it will be difficult to respond quickly to someone charging you from the side, trying to knock you over); too much SNS activity can inhibit performance, causing an increase in errors or poor accuracy. While an athlete can perform in a situation that feels threatening, for optimal performance, the interaction between the athlete and the environment should be positive (Hanin 2000). Fortunately, as teachers, we can provide an environment that feels safe, increasing the likelihood of the student's ability to learn.

A new movement in a new environment can be experienced in many ways. How the teacher introduces the movement can be the difference between a successful experience and one that is perceived as negative. Imagine a new student begins seeing you for movement education. She announces in the initial visit that she has knee pain that gets worse when she tries to squat. She has a small meniscus tear in her left knee that she is sure is the cause of her pain. What are some things that will reduce her sense of safety?

If you, the teacher, argue with her about her ability to squat, that will make her defensive and she will feel threatened. This will heighten her SNS response and make it difficult for her to execute tasks related to squatting in an efficient way, potentially making her pain worse. Another strategy that would reduce her sense of safety would be having her squat. Because she perceives squatting to be a painful activity, asking her to do the very thing she just told you causes pain will decrease her confidence in you and make her feel like the environment, and you as a teacher, aren't safe.

What could you do instead to make her feel both safe and capable?

Rather than asking her to squat, you could place her in positions that resemble a squat and assess how she feels. For instance, you might ask her to lie down on her back and place her feet on a wall so her knees are bent to a 90° angle. If this doesn't cause pain, you could have her press her feet into the wall in different ways, creating a connection between her feet and the muscles that activate in her legs and hips. Maybe you eventually have her lie down on a blanket so when she presses her feet into the wall, her body moves away from the wall, resembling a squat on her back.

Or maybe you have her come into a seated position with her feet flat on the floor and you ask her to press her feet into the ground, cueing different aspects of the feet to press into until she begins to feel the muscles supporting her in her legs and hips. Over time, as she gains confidence pressing into her feet, you might ask her to press into her feet until her hips come off the seat, floating right above the seat. Eventually, she may press into her feet, float her hips,

press into her feet more, and stand all the way up, reversing the process on the way down. Why would these scenarios potentially work?

When you place the person in a position that doesn't cause discomfort, the nervous system relaxes. Usually, lying on the back with the feet on the wall can be done in such a way that it is comfortable. Sitting can also usually be done in a way that feels comfortable, as long as the teacher is open minded, listens to the student, and makes the appropriate modifications to enhance the student's comfort, such as raising the height of the seat or changing the foot or pelvis position. Focusing the student's attention on the kinesthetic and interoceptive sensations of the feet and the muscular effort involved introduces a strategy in a position that resembles the bottom of the squat but doesn't involve "work" in the knees, influencing the core response network (CRN).

The core response network is comprised of the ANS, the emotional motor system, the reticular arousal system, and the limbic system to organize immediate, instinctive responses to environmental challenges before conscious processing (Payne et al. 2015). The ANS, remember, is the autonomic nervous system and can either calm things down through a PNS response or amp things up via an SNS response.

The emotional motor system (EMS) is comprised of sub-cortical motor centers and causes emotion-specific movements and postures to occur outside of voluntary control. Have you ever noticed someone clenching their jaw before they do a lunge movement or tightening three fingers before lifting a leg? Those are unconscious movements happening at the behest of the EMS.

The reticular arousal system (RAS) controls alertness and orientation. It plays a role in determining where your attention is focused and how much arousal is needed in the moment. Hyper-vigilance causes upregulation of the RAS while hypo-vigilance causes decreased RAS output. The RAS plays an important role in the sleep–wake cycle and the startle response (the initial response that occurs when you hear a loud sound or are caught off guard). Arousal is necessary for learning; too much arousal inhibits learning, so the goal becomes finding the optimal level of arousal for the task (Skinner et al. 2004).

The limbic system (LS) includes the hippocampus, amygdala, and septal regions of the brain. It is responsible for recalling emotionally significant events and is central to fear- and pleasure-based experiences. Emotion plays a strong role in learning and memory; the hippocampus plays a critical role in long-term memory storage, while the amygdala helps consolidate and retrieve emotional memories (Rajmohan & Mohandas 2007). In a learning environment, the emotional response of the student will partially determine how the information is received and, ultimately, whether it's retained.

All of these systems work together to allow the CRN to respond quickly, with little conscious consideration, to stimuli that is potentially threatening or arousing. This informs a person's neuroceptive state.

If the student who is scared to squat because it causes her pain is asked to squat without any alternative sensory experiences explored, several unconscious kinesthetic and interoceptive cues occur, causing her to move in a way that reinforces a painful experience. Because the movement doesn't feel safe to her, an unconscious chain of reactions influences her motor patterns and experience. The experience and CRN are altered when she is placed in alternative positions, creating a less threatening, safer view and, it is hoped, a different response when she eventually tries the squatting pattern.

Case study

Recently, I was teaching my husband a different way to perform a front roll. He did Aikido for a while, and front rolls used to bother his left shoulder and chest area. As I watched him roll over his left side, I noticed his left shoulder twitched up just as he was getting ready to roll over it. This happened every time he rolled over that side. The movement of rolling was coupled with the movement of tensing the shoulder. He broke left collarbone several years ago. The break required surgery and he had never been quite as comfortable on that side afterwards.

Feldenkrais, a mind–body movement modality based on conscious movement and finding ease and fluidity, was developed by Moshé Feldenkrais. Remember how I talked about the EMS causing emotion-specific movements outside of conscious control? Feldenkrais called these types of movements parasitic movements. Another

way to think of these pairings is that they are movement habits, attached to unconscious emotions. In my husband's case, the stimulus of rolling over the left shoulder triggered a response of hiking the left shoulder up. The left shoulder hike does nothing to help the roll, and as soon as it was brought to his attention, he consciously changed how he rolled and it felt immediately better. As soon as he stopped thinking about it, he reverted back to hiking his shoulder. Habits, as you learned earlier, are hard to break because breaking them requires conscious effort. Can my husband change his rolling pattern so it no longer involves a left shoulder hike? Yes, but it will take breaking down the pattern, focusing his attention, and practicing rolling in a variety of ways until not hiking his shoulder becomes an automatic response and he moves into the autonomous phase of learning.

Attention, neuroception, and mindful movement

Open monitoring

Another form of paying attention is open monitoring. It's a common meditation technique that involves observing without judgment. It's noticing your environment, you in your environment, and what you are feeling without trying to change anything. When you ask yourself, "How am I feeling?" you are performing open monitoring.

What open monitoring *isn't* is blaming. When someone arrives for a session and tells you their transverse abdominis isn't firing and that's why their sacrum is unstable, that isn't open monitoring. That is assigning a cause, judging a physical sensation, and creating a threat response around a body part, in this case, the sacrum. If the student were to walk in and say instead, "I feel a sensation of looseness in my low back" this is an observation. The CRN will respond differently to the second statement than the first. Observation implies something can change, that learning can take place, and the situation is temporary. Judging has a more permanent feeling to it and is related to a fixed mindset, eliminating the possibility of change.

In the book, *Buddha's brain: The practical neuroscience of happiness, love & wisdom,* author and neuropsychologist Rick Hanson explains that the more you make associations between a behavior and a feeling, the more likely the behavior will evoke the feeling. It's how learning in general happens – your brain knows when this happens, then that happens. When learning becomes autonomous, there is no conscious effort required to make the connections – you just know the outcome based on previously learned experiences. As you have seen, sometimes these unconscious, learned motor patterns become obsolete and no longer necessary to perform a specific task well. Teaching people to be more conscious of their movements by asking them what they are feeling can break automatic behaviors by interrupting patterns that are on autopilot (Hanson & Mendius 2009).

When people are told specific movements are "bad" or that certain muscles "aren't working," they adopt movement strategies that reflect their beliefs. If someone assumes bending over is bad for their back because one time they forgot to squat down and felt something in their back that they associated with pain, and they have been told by authorities that picking something up wrong will ruin their back, then every time they bend over in a way they deem "wrong," their CRN would cause a subtle bracing action, preparing for the inevitable threat they associate with the movement. When they experience the pain they anticipate, they think "Aha! I knew bending over was bad for my back." The association is reinforced with each subsequent "faulty" bending pattern until, eventually, they wouldn't bend over at all, creating stiffness and rigidity in the spine and creating an internal narrative that bending over equals back pain.

If, instead, they changed their internal dialog to, "My spine is strong and resilient. It can withstand lots of load. When I bend over, I am going to observe what I experience, and if I sense discomfort, I am going to try bending in a different way," their attitude about their back would change. They would no longer judge the movement of bending as good or bad, or equate the movement of bending with back pain. By using a growth mindset and open monitoring during a movement they have sensitivity around, they are able to learn how to bend in a way that feels better while cultivating a more curious inner narrative.

This is a technique I frequently use when I work with individuals with low back pain. I have found that if the expectation is that bending over will hurt, the first time it will probably hurt; but if I ask the person to do it again, a little bit slower and they don't go down as far, chances are high that it won't hurt. And if they do it a third time and a fourth time, they usually find that it gets easier, and their fear begins to subside. I usually have the client stop after the fourth or fifth time, so they end on a positive note, and then have them try it again, in a slightly different way, the next time I see them.

You can also shift the student's focus, cueing the movement task as a combination of open monitoring and focused attention. Ask how they are performing the movement. Can they do it a little bit differently? How does that feel? Can they think about reaching the arms down, or feeling the ribs flex, or leading with the eyes? How do those variations feel? Ask the student to be an observer of the experience, almost like they are watching a movie and not judging or assigning phrases like "bad," "harmful," or "likely to cause catastrophic injury." Sometimes the teacher's job is to ask questions, not provide the answers.

Open monitoring can also be translated as being present. An easy way to practice this is during walks outside.

Practical application

Go for a 10- to 20-minute walk outside. Once every couple of minutes, feel the air against your skin. Listen to the sound of your feet against the ground. Listen to the sound of your breath. Look around you and see what you see. After your check-in, return to your thoughts and repeat the awareness exercise again, a few minutes later.

At the end of your walk, take a moment to assess your current state. How do you feel? Energized? More alert? More present?

Encouraging students to regularly participate in cardiovascular exercise outside can double as a way for them to practice open monitoring. Not only is cardiovascular activity good for the heart, it reduces blood sugar and pain symptoms (Ambrose & Golightly 2015). It can also act as a form of moving meditation. Open monitoring techniques have a host of benefits, including:

- improved feelings of well-being and happiness
- improved creativity (Fujino et al. 2018; Colzato et al. 2012)
- decreased feelings of anxiety
- decreased feelings of depression
- decreased stress
- reduced experience of pain (Zeidan & Vago 2018).

Interspersing open monitoring during an activity that doesn't require a lot of focus is a great way to practice the concept of mindful movement. Mindful movement can be defined as movement that involves the interaction between mind, body, and behavior. Modalities that require either focused attention or use open monitoring can be considered mindful movement (Hwan et al. 2013). Most movement skills can be performed in a way that employs an element of mindfulness, as you saw with both the squatting walking examples earlier.

Mindful movement

Modern mind–body movement training likely has its roots in ancient Greek culture. Early documentation of Western mind–body exercise philosophy suggests it was created by Pehr Henrik Ling, the father of Swedish gymnastics, in the late eighteenth century (Hoffman & Gabel 2016). From 1890 to 1925, six mind–body methods emerged, sharing similar philosophies and based on similar exercises. They all emphasized the utilization of bodyweight exercises, breathing, and creating a mind–body connection through conscious awareness.

Creating conscious awareness of how the body moves disrupts the CRN and requires focused attention, at least initially. As the skill becomes autonomous, the attention can shift, becoming more of an inquiry. Mindful movement can be used to finesse small movements, which you will experience in some of the exercises depicted below. It can also be used to perform bigger, more integrative movements such as climbing a tree or balancing a dowel on your hand while you kneel down and come back to a standing position. It could be argued that even larger, power-based movements have an element of mindfulness. Have you ever tried to clean a barbell that's heavier than you are used to or performed a series of kettlebell swings, alternating between two hands and one hand in a rhythmic way? There is an element of focus required, as well as the constant monitoring of tension and ease. Challenge is what creates an opportunity for learning. Challenge, it turns out, can take on a variety of forms, from the subtle to the complex.

Exercise
Focusing the eyes

Come into a comfortable seated position. Focus your eyes on something that is near you. Now, focus your eyes on something that is far away from you. Go back and forth between the objects 8–10 times.

Now, focus your eyes on something that is near you but slightly to the left. Now, look at something that is far away from you and slightly to the right. Go back and forth between the objects 8–10 times.

Finally, look at something that is near you, but slightly to the right. Now, look at something that is far away and slightly to the left. Go back and forth between the objects 8–10 times.

Questions to consider and observe

- Did the neck move? Could it be done without the neck moving?
- What about the jaw? Did it move? If so, could it be done without the jaw moving?
- How did it feel? Were the objects clear or blurry?
- Did you remember to breathe?

Exercise
Centering from the feet

Set a timer for 60 seconds. Come into a standing position. Close your eyes. Take a minute to observe the environment, the texture of the floor against the feet, the ambient temperature of the room, and the sounds around you.

When the timer goes off, open your eyes. Begin lifting the inside of your right foot off of the

ground. Feel the outer edge of the right foot against the ground. Repeat this 10 times and switch sides (Figure 4.1).

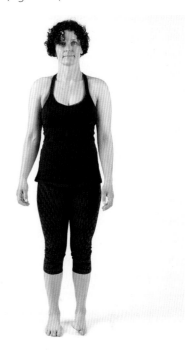

Figure 4.1

Now, lift the outer edge of the right foot off of the ground. Feel the inside edge of the right foot against the ground. Lower the outer edge of the right foot down and repeat the movement 10 times.

Lift the right heel off of the floor. Feel the weight of the right forefoot against the ground. Set the heel down. Repeat 10 times and switch sides.

Lift the right front of the foot off of the floor. Feel the weight of the heel against the floor and set it down. Repeat 10 times.

Finally, lift the right foot off the ground. Set it down and feel the weight of the right foot against the ground as you lift the left foot off of the ground. Go back and forth between the feet 10 times.

Come back up into a quiet standing position. Set a timer for 1 minute. Take one more minute to close your eyes and observe what you feel, sense, and hear. When the timer goes off, open your eyes.

Questions to consider and observe

- Did you feel yourself moving a lot when your eyes were closed?

- Was your experience of observing different between the first minute and the second minute? If so, how?

Exercise
The upper body in space

Come into a seated position with the arms resting by the sides. Let the arms and hands rest in a comfortable position.

Set a timer for 1 minute. Close your eyes and observe your body. Notice what sensations you are feeling, the temperature of the room against your skin, and any discomfort. If you feel any discomfort, observe it curiously, without assigning blame or any negativity to it.

When the timer goes off, open your eyes. Keep your feet in contact with the floor and rest the arms by your sides. Imagine the arms are heavy. It's as though they each weigh 20 kg (45 lb).

Now, lift the heavy arms up. Feel how hard it is to lift them. When you can't lift them any higher because they are so heavy, let them drop down. Do this three times.

Let go of the idea that your arms are heavy. Take a moment to feel how the arms are resting by your side. Can you feel their weight?

Now, imagine someone is standing in front of you, and the person has taken hold of your hands and is lifting them up for you. Let the imaginary person lift the arms to shoulder height or slightly above, and then let the imaginary person lower your arms down. Do this three times.

Sit with your arms long. Feel how they are hanging. How does that feel?

Imagine there is an object in front of you, just out of your reach, that you want. Reach the arms up and toward the object. Really try to reach the object. Lower the arms down. Do this three times.

Sit with the arms long. Feel the arms and how they hang in space, and feel how the fingers are an extension of the hand.

Set a timer for 1 minute. Close your eyes, and observe your body and the space around your body. If you come across sensations that draw your attention, take a moment to recognize them, acknowledge them, and return to observing your body and the space around you.

Questions to consider

- Did the different lifting conditions (arms heavy, someone lifting them for you, reaching), change your experience of lifting the arms? If so, how?

- Which condition did you like the best? Why?

- If you felt sensations when you were practicing open monitoring, were you able to just note the sensations, or did you find yourself wanting to assign words to the sensations?

- Did your mind wander during the two separate minutes? If so, did you catch your mind wandering and bring it back to the task at hand or did you let it wander?

All of these exercises use either focused attention or open monitoring to establish a connection between different aspects of the physical body and the mind. Before you move on, read through the exercises again and identify when open monitoring is being used and when focused attention is being used.

These types of exercises teach the basic principles of meditation through movement. Occasionally, rather than moving, the student is asked to sit quietly and observe. This gives the student an opportunity to observe and reflect.

Not everyone responds to sitting quietly, just like not everyone responds to moving the entire time. Gauge the student and their level of focus. For students with a lot of energy, teaching open monitoring toward the end of their session or asking questions about their observations throughout the session can introduce this form of meditation to the student in a more accessible way.

The value of words

The way humans communicate is through language, both body language and actual words. One way to help people establish a mind–body connection is to ask them to describe how they are doing an action with their body or to describe their experience of performing the specific task.

One of the areas of the brain that controls movement, the motor cortex, is activated when a word is said or read (de Lafuente & Romo 2004). This means when someone says the word "jump," the motor cortex plans how it would jump. Because the brain has a clear picture of what jumping means, it can plan accordingly. When you, the teacher, use a word the student doesn't understand, an accurate image of the motor skill can't be clearly constructed by the motor cortex. (Have you ever asked someone who hasn't exercised in 30 years to do a squat? I have, and let's just say their idea of what a squat looks like and my idea of what a squat looks like differ.) Asking people to use their words also focuses their attention on what they were doing and forces them to recall how they performed the action, which assists with learning (Chatterjee 2010).

The ability to articulate how the body moves creates a sense of ownership and autonomy around movement. It decreases the chasm between the mind and the body as separate entities and begins to unify them.

Another benefit of paying attention to how daily movements are performed is that it creates an opportunity to explore how the same action could be done differently. One of my favorite games to play during my own personal workout is "What happens if …?" What happens if I angle my fingers a slightly differently way when I handstand? What happens if I pay attention to gripping the bar as hard as I can during my deadlifts? What happens

if I think about moving different parts of my spine up toward the ceiling when I do spinal warm-ups? What happens if I initiate rolling from the pelvis instead of my feet? You get the idea.

It can be more subtle, as well. What happens if I reach with my right hand instead of my left for the glass? What happens if I interlock my fingers in the way that feels awkward and reach them out in front of me?

I often ask clients, "What are you experiencing?" or "Can you tell me how you are doing that?" People who aren't used to describing their movements often visibly squirm. When there is a disconnect between the mind and the body, it's uncomfortable to try to articulate what the body is doing. The inability to use words to describe physical movements impacts perception and experience.

With practice, the ability to put words to the physical experience becomes easier. Words create a bridge between thinking about an action and actually performing the action. Words can make movement more mindful.

Neuroception, focused attention, and open monitoring are foundations for learning. In order to be effective as a teacher, it's important to ask yourself, "How can I make the process of learning most accessible for my student? Do they struggle with focus? Do they trust their body is capable of supporting them during the skill I am about to ask them to do? If not, how can I make the skill feel safer? Where do I need to add more support? Can the student observe what they are experiencing?" We will return to these concepts as we further explore the idea of learning as it relates to specific areas in the next chapters.

References

Ambrose KR and Golightly YM (2015) Physical exercise as a non-pharmacological treatment of pain: Why and when. Best Practice & Research. Clinical Pharmacology 29 (1) 120–130.

Chan RW, Lushington K, and Immink MA (2018) States of focused attention and sequential action: A comparison of single session meditation and computerized attention task influences on top-down control during sequence learning. Acta Psychiatrica Scandinavica 191 87–100.

Chatterjee A (2010) Disembodying cognition. Language and Cognition 2 (1) 79–116.

Chua LK, Dimpapilis MK, Iwatsuki T, Abdollahipour R, Lewthaite R, and Wulf G (2019) Practice variability promotes an external focus of attention and enhances motor learning. Human Movement Science 64 307–319.

Colzato LS, Ozturk A, and Hommel B (2012) Meditate to create: The impact of focused-attention and open monitoring training on convergent and divergent thinking. Frontiers in Psychology 3 116.

de Lafuente V and Romo R (2004) Language abilities of motor cortex. Neuron 41 (2) 178–180.

Fujino M, Ueda Y, Mizuhara H, Saiki J, and Ndmura M (2018) Open monitoring meditation reduces the involvement of brain regions related to memory function. Scientific Reports 8 (9,968).

Hanin YL (ed.) (2000) Emotions in sport. Champaign, IL: Human Kinetics.

Hanson R and Mendius R (2009) Buddha's brain: The practical neuroscience of happiness, love & wisdom. Oakland, CA: New Harbinger Publications.

Hoffman J and Gabel CP (2016) The origins of Western mind–body exercise methods. Physical Therapy Reviews 20 (5–6) 315–324.

Hwan Kim S, Schneider SM, Kravitz L, Mermier C, and Burge MR (2013) Mind–body practices for post-traumatic stress disorder. Journal of Investigative Medicine 61 (5) 827–834.

Luque D (2017) Goal-directed and habit-like modulations of stimulus processing during reinforcement learning. The Journal of Neuroscience 37 (11) 3,009–3,017.

Morasso P, Casadio M, Mohan V, Rea F, and Zenzen J (2015) Revisiting the body-schema concept in the context of whole-body postural-focal dynamics. Frontiers in Human Neuroscience 9 83.

Oppezzo M and Schwartz DL (2014) Give your ideas some legs: The positive effect of walking on creative thinking. Journal of Experimental Psychology: Learning, Memory, and Cognition 40 (4) 1,142–1,152.

Payne P, Levine PA, and Crane-Godreau MA (2015) Somatic experiencing: Using interoception and proprioception as core elements of trauma therapy. Frontiers in Psychology 6 93.

Pollack CL, Boyd LA, Hunt MA, and Garland J (2014) Use of the challenge point framework to guide motor learning of stepping reactions for improved balance control in people with stroke: A case series. Physical Therapy 94 (4) 562–570.

Porges SW (2009) The polyvagal theory: New insights into adaptive reactions of the autonomic nervous system. Cleveland Clinic Journal of Medicine 76 (2) 86–90.

Rajmohan V and Mohandas E (2007) The limbic system. Indian Journal of Psychiatry 49 (2) 132–139.

Ramirez-Vizcaya S and Froese T (2019) The enactive approach to habits: New concepts for the cognitive science of bad habits and addiction. Frontiers in Psychology 10 301.

Sbardelotto ML, Costa RR, Malysz KA, Pedroso GS, Pereira BC, Sorato HR, Silvera PCL, Nesi RT, Grande AJ, and Pinho RA (2019) Improvement in muscular strength and aerobic capacities in elderly people occurs independently of physical training type or exercise model. Clinics (Sao Paulo) 74 e833.

Skinner RD, Homma Y, and Garcia-Rill E (2004) Arousal mechanisms related to posture and loco-motion: 2. Ascending modulation. Progress in Brain Research 143 291–298.

Taylor JA and Ivry RB (2015) The roles of strategies in motor learning. Annals of the New York Academy of Sciences 1,251 1–12.

Wood W and Runger D (2016) Psychology of habit. Annual Review of Psychology 67 289–314.

Wulf G (2007) Attention and motor skill learning. Champaign, IL: Human Kinetics.

Yeung N and Monsell S (2003) Switching between tasks of unequal familiarity: The role of stimulus-attribute and response-set selection. Journal of Experimental Pychology: Human Perception & Performance 29 (2) 455–469.

Zeidan F and Vago D (2018) Mindfulness-based pain relief: A mechanistic account. Annals of the New York Academy of Sciences 1,373 (1) 114–127.

Case study

A client was referred to me who had been experiencing neck pain. She wanted to get stronger and fitter, but was worried about injuring herself in a traditional exercise setting.

As I watched her move, I noticed she didn't use her feet to engage with the ground. They weren't responsive to her movements, and she never used the entire foot – it was almost like the middle of the foot hovered off the floor, never quite making contact with the floor beneath her.

I began bringing her attention to her feet and how she used them, offering cues to help her integrate them more during specific movements. When she left after that first session, she later told me, she went to her car and cried. She could feel her feet in a way that she hadn't in a long time and she felt hopeful that she could move through her neck pain. (She saw me for about four months, her neck pain disappeared, and she was able to get back to the activities she enjoyed.)

What do the neck and the feet have to do with each other, you might be wondering? This chapter includes a brief overview of how the vestibular system and the visual system work, where they are located (hint: they are connected to the same area in which the client was experiencing pain), and how the feet are a major component to maintaining balance. If you take the feet away as a source of information to the nervous system, the primary sources of information left to help maintain balance are located in the eyes and ears, which are located on the skull, which is connected to the neck. When the other balance systems of the body are working extra hard to maintain balance, especially the visual system, the neck muscles sometimes work harder than they need to in order to maintain a sense of stability and safety. When attention is focused to the foot, the nervous system suddenly receives afferent information from a different source, increasing safety and stability, and allowing more balance between the SNS and the PNS. The neck

muscles, which are involved both in accessory breathing strategies during the fight-or-flight response and when the eyes are being heavily relied upon for input, are finally able to relax. The entire body, from head to toes, works in a more integrated way when the neuromuscular system has sensory input from a spectrum of sources.

The feet are important body parts. When you ask students to describe how the foot interacts with the ground, unless their feet hurt or they have gone down the rabbit hole of foot health and strength because something specific piqued their curiosity, chances are high they will pause, searching for the words to describe their feet because they haven't thought much about them in a long time. When people lack kinesthetic awareness of the feet, they are missing huge amounts of sensory information from the afferent nervous system, influencing proprioception. Since the feet provide a stable support to maintain balance and propel the body forward, this lack of kinesthetic and proprioceptive awareness decreases balance security and safety.

As you will see throughout the chapter, the foot acts like a spring to propel you forward. The sensory receptors throughout the foot and ankle tell the neuromuscular system about the type of surface you are on, whether you have enough support under the feet to feel stable, and whether the feet are on a surface that is slanted or flat. All of this information informs balance and stability. Balance is defined as an even distribution of weight that allows someone to stay upright and steady, or stable. Remember, stability is the ability to recover from perturbations, so another way to think of balance when you are considering the feet is that it's the ability of the feet to feel connected to the ground in a way that will allow them to respond and recover from potential perturbations. (We will discuss this further in Chapter 6.) Balance is determined primarily by three systems mentioned above: the vestibular system, the visual system, and the proprioceptive system.

continued

The vestibular system is located in the inner ear and is possibly the most ancient sensory system in vertebrates – balance is that important (Highstein 2004). It gives sensory feedback about angular and linear movement of the head. Because the head rarely comes into contact with the ground, there's less sensory feedback from pressure on the skin to inform the proprioceptive system about its location. Since the skull houses the brain, knowing where the head is oriented is critical for maintaining a sense of safety. Keeping the head upright is one of the first things babies learn how to do, and the vestibular system plays an important role in maintaining balance.

If the vestibular system isn't working properly, it can wreak havoc on proprioception, interoception, and a general sense of well-being. When one of the crystals that sits on the hair of the inner ear, whose job is to inform the vestibular system about position, gets knocked loose, the neuromuscular system is sent into a tizzy. The vestibular system stops receiving accurate information, creating a situation that is akin to perpetual seasickness. This is also one of the causes of vertigo, a word used to describe the sensation of spinning and loss of balance.

Vertigo can also be triggered by changing the direction of the head too quickly. Have you ever gotten on a swing as an adult and begun pumping your legs, expecting to find the thrill of flying like you did as a child, only to discover you were left with the distinct feeling of dizziness and nausea? As a child, you practice changing your head and body position regularly. In fact, it's almost like children crave vestibular input. They play games that spin them around in circles like Ring Around the Rosie; they want the adults in their life to throw them in the air; and they play on playground equipment that involves swinging, climbing, and spinning. In a children's world, roller coasters are fun, and a fast change in direction is welcomed; adults, on the other hand, often find themselves politely declining anything that triggers a rapid change in position for fear it will cause the overwhelming sensation of nausea (or trigger an actual reaction that involves regurgitation).

Like many things, the sensation of vertigo can be lessened if students are exposed gradually to movements that require a change in head position. If people participate entirely in movements that require linear movements, their vestibular systems won't be accustomed to dealing with the stress and challenge of changing positions quickly. Unless your students participate in hobbies like martial arts or Parkour, or they happen to work at an amusement park where they ride roller coasters for fun, introducing movements that require a change in head position should be done slowly, giving the system time to adapt.

Training the vestibular system in a progressive way creates adaptability and better equips students for balance challenges (Han et al. 2011). One of the ways to train the vestibular system is to train the second system that determines balance: the eyes.

The visual system, along with the vestibular system, orients people to their surroundings. Their eyes take in input from the environment and let the brain know where they are located in relation to objects in the physical world. When the eyes perceive a situation that's potentially threatening, it can cause feelings of nausea, similar to the feeling of nausea that happens when adults try swinging for the first time in fifteen years. The nauseous feeling is an interoceptive sense triggered by the visual system. Have you ever stood at the edge of the Grand Canyon and looked down, pondering what would happen if the rail around the rim gave way? The sensation of nausea and dizziness that waves over you is the physiological response to a situation that could be perceived as dangerous, based on information from the visual system.

Though the eyes are important for balance, it's possible to balance without the eyes, albeit with a little less stability. Try this: stand up. Look straight ahead and feel how much your body is swaying. Is it a lot or a little?

continued

Now, close your eyes. Try not to change your head position. Notice how much your body is swaying. Is it more or less than when your eyes were open?

Most people notice themselves swaying more when their eyes are closed than when they are open. Take away one system, and another system has to work a bit harder. In this case, the system that kicks in to make up for the loss of the visual system is the third system used to determine balance: the proprioceptive system.

We discussed proprioception in depth in Chapter 2; we also discussed the importance of body schema and how it affects a person's perception of self and movement in Chapter 1. Think back to the homunculus man I mentioned. Which body parts tend to be exaggerated? The tongue, the hands, and the feet. Why? Because these areas take up large amounts of space in the motor cortex. The hands and tongue must be able to perform small movements for fine motor tasks such as typing, grasping, talking, and eating. I mentioned earlier that the feet and ankle are filled with proprioceptors to maintain a sense of balance and stability during dynamic tasks. Here's the interesting thing about proprioception: while there are nerves throughout the body that contain mechanoreceptors, the control of upright posture is heavily dependent on the mechanoreceptors detecting limb position in the lower extremities (van Deursen & Simoneau 1999). Ankle proprioception, specifically, enables the foot to make small adjustments and maintain balance while the upper body moves (Han et al. 2015). Another way to look at this is that the feet and ankles provide the information the neuromuscular system needs in order to stay upright, moving, and balanced in a wide range of positions. The accuracy of the information and whether the neuromuscular system feels safe is reliant on awareness, mobility, and strength of the feet and ankles.

When you think about the fact that two-thirds of the information related to balance comes from the head (the inner ears and the eyes), the sensory information the feet and ankles provides is important because it is input from the only part of the body actually in contact with the ground. The amount of information the nervous system can detect from the feet and their contact with the ground is impressive and impacts proprioceptive feedback and kinesthetic awareness throughout the lower limb. What happens at the feet can affect what happens at the knees, which can affect what happens at the hips, which can affect what happens at the back. (The reverse is also true. If you shift the position of your pelvis you can change how the foot is pressing into the ground. We'll talk about that more later.)

However, the feet are often shod, to protect them from hard, manmade surfaces that are consistent in texture and hardness. The feet conform to the environment in which they spend the most time, so stable soles and shoes reduce the foot's mobility and prevent it from relying on muscular strength to propel the body forward. The result is that the shoe that provides stability creates a foot that is stiff and weak.

When the foot and ankle aren't used on a variety of surfaces regularly, they become less adaptable. The ankle's ability to respond to terrain that is varied decreases; the modern-day solution to this is to place the ankle in boots to create ankle stability and reduce the risk of the ankle deviating from its position, ultimately creating an ankle that lacks controlled strength. (Or mobility, depending on how you look at it.) Ankle supports, inserts, and braces can be a good, temporary solution when immobilization is required because of injury, but if the goal is to create a strong and mobile structure that is responsive to the ground, provides accurate information to the neuromuscular system, and is accurately depicted in the body schema, the foot and ankle should be trained like any other body part: progressively and in a variety of ways, to improve resilience and function.

continued

Chapter 5

Case study *continued*

The toes, the digits of the lower extremity that provide balance and support to the foot, often become curled, taking the shape of the shoe (Hughes et al. 1990). Even when they don't become curled, there is frequently a disconnect between the toes and the neuromuscular system, leading to a lack of conscious control of toe movement. It's funny, but when you don't see a specific body part, it's easy to "forget" the area moves, or that you can ask the area to move. As noted in Chapter 2, the less in touch you are with various body parts, the fuzzier their image will be in your mind's eye. The big toe (or the great toe, as it is often called), helps propel the foot forward during walking and helps maintain balance (Chou et al. 2009). It can be moved independently from the other toes and ideally should be able to actively press into the ground, creating a stable platform for propulsion. The toes are important, but often neglected because of fashion matters; taking a genuine interest in how people use their ankles, feet, and toes can enhance efficiency and balance and improve their sense of safety.

Changing how the body is used by altering perception causes the loads on the musculoskeletal system to shift. This, in turn, changes the feedback the brain receives from the afferent nervous system. The beauty of this is that sometimes a subtle shift is all the nervous system needs to change the sensation of tightness, stiffness, or discomfort. Because the feet are so sensory rich, focusing attention through cueing or somatic-based exercises can trigger a profound shift throughout the body.

Exercise
Sensing the toes and the feet

Come into a comfortable seated position on the floor. Close your eyes and imagine your feet. How much of them can you sense? Is one foot bigger than the other?

Now, if you are wearing shoes, take them off and return to your seated position. Set a timer for 1 minute. Cross your right ankle over your left knee so you can get a hold of your right foot. Bend it, twist it, press on it. Tug on your toes. Massage different points of the foot. When the timer goes off, switch sides, spending 1 minute doing the same thing with the left foot.

When you have finished re-acquainting yourself with your feet, close your eyes and imagine your feet. Do they feel different than they did when you were standing on them before you spent time touching them? Is your image of them more or less clear?

I already discussed how touch is an effective way to improve body image. When you ask people to touch and manipulate their feet, it improves the accuracy of the body schema by reinforcing the fact that the feet are a part of the body. The hands are doing the sensing, so information about the hands is also getting sent to the somatic branch of the nervous system, creating a connection between the feet, the hands, and how they relate to each other within the internal body map. This technique of touching various areas seems to be particularly effective at establishing connections for people who struggle with feeling specific parts of their body. If a student has ever said to you, "It doesn't feel like my foot/hand/shoulder/knee," touching the foot/hand/shoulder knee reassures them that, indeed, that specific body part really is a part of them.

The anatomy of the foot

The foot is an intricately designed structure. There are 26 bones in the feet and 34 synovial joints, 18 of which are curved (Ridola et al. 2007). There are four layers of muscle and three layers of ligaments, which bind together with the tendons to hold the foot bones in an arched position, while still allowing the foot to have mobility and springiness (Wright et al. 2012). There are several nerves innervating the foot, allowing the foot to interact with the ground and detect changes in pressure and surface. Numerous somatosensory receptors are located in the ligaments that comprise the foot arch, joint capsules, intrinsic foot muscles, and mechanoreceptors of the sole of the foot.

The foot is designed to be flexible, allowing the arch to flatten as it responds to the ground, which creates the elastic energy storage in the longitudinal arch that propels you forward. It's also designed to be strong, so the arch doesn't collapse to the floor during quiet standing. These two functions, serving as a lever to propel the body forward during running and walking and supporting the weight of the body, are both dynamic in nature since, as discussed earlier, the body is never truly still.

The tibiotalar joint is primarily how the foot points and extends or, more technically, plantar flexes and dorsiflexes. There is a junction between the talus and the navicular bones called the transverse tarsal joint. The talus is the small bone that sits between the heel bone and the two bones of the lower leg, the tibia and fibula. It works with the subtalar joint to allow the arch of the foot to flatten and dome, depending on the stage of the gait cycle. The foot flattens as the body moves over it, storing the elastic energy needed to dome and propel the leg forward. The flattening and the doming of the foot are complex, three-dimensional movements that are also referred to as pronation and supination, respectively (Rockar 1995).

Because the talus articulates with the tibia, it serves as a connection point between the foot and the lower leg at the tibiotalar joint (don't worry, there won't be a test on all of these terms later). Understanding the complexity of the anatomy gives you the chance to appreciate how intricate and dynamic the movements are that allow you to move forward, with every step.

The movement of the heel complements the movement of the midfoot. The inside of the heel can move closer to the ground, which it does during ankle eversion, or farther away from the ground, which it does during ankle inversion. (If you really want to make your brain tired, another way to think about this is the outside of the heel comes farther away from the ground during eversion and closer to the ground during inversion.) These movements are generally fairly small, and there are several ligaments that support the ankle and prevent excess mobility at the joint (Brockett & Chapman 2016).

As you walk, the heel rolls in (everts) and the arch flattens (pronates) so force can be absorbed. These movements are also small, controlled by the fascia, muscles, ligaments, and tendons that comprise the arch. As you get ready to toe off and swing the leg forward, the big toe extends and pushes down, causing the foot to become rigid. The arch stiffens (supinates) and the ankle moves out, or inverts, creating a stiff platform and allowing you to push off on a strong lever (Chan & Rudins 1994).

Practical application

Before you read any further, set a timer for 3 minutes. Based on your understanding of supination, pronation, inversion, and eversion, play with these concepts in a variety of positions. For instance, you can perform eversion supine, in an open-chain position, or with your knee bent. You can do the same movement with your knee straight or with your heel resting on the floor. How many variations can you come up with?

Research suggests one of the best ways to truly understand a topic is to test yourself on the concepts (Lang 2016). In movement sciences, one way to test yourself on the concepts is to isolate the movement you are learning and applying it across a wide spectrum of positions. It's okay if you don't "get it" right away. With time, practice, and repeated exposure, isolated movements and how they integrate with the rest of the body will become clearer.

Another way to create mobility and stability through the foot and ankle is to walk over varied terrain. When the ground isn't perfectly even, the feet are required to make small adjustments, adapting to the surface beneath them, which strengthens the feet at a variety of angles. Not everyone has access to hiking trails or beaches, and that's okay. The exercises throughout the rest of this chapter are designed to create a better sense of awareness of the feet, helping students more clearly feel the feet and understand how they work by using a variety of positions and tools. The exercises can be implemented as neuromuscular/motor control warm-ups before dynamic balance or strength-based work such as deadlifts or squats. If you are sequencing a class around single-leg balance, adding in exercises such as the ones found below can prime the student's neuromuscular system for the task and create more efficient options for balancing on one foot.

Exercise

Sensing the position of the feet

With bare feet, come into a standing position, with your hands by your side and your weight in your feet. Without looking at your feet, can you bring the big toes together so they are touching? How does that feel?

Now, separate the feet a little bit and turn the toes out. Try to turn the toes out the same amount. Give yourself a few seconds in that position before you look down and check your foot position. Are your feet even? Are your toes angled out at the same angle?

Try turning your toes in at the same angle. How does that feel? Are your feet turned in the same amount? Look down and check.

Finally, move your feet to their comfortable resting place. How does that feel? Glance down and see if your feet are even or if one foot is back, a little bit out, or a little bit in. If it is, don't try to change anything. Just notice what you find comfortable.

Knowing where the feet are in relation to each other when they are on the ground is important for kinesthetic awareness and proprioception of the lower extremities. A number of factors can influence the accuracy of the perception of the feet, including injuries at the hip joint, injury at the knee joint, laxity of ligaments in the lower extremities, previous trauma to the lower extremities or feet, and the ever-common ankle sprain.

Ankle sprains usually happen when the heel inverts more than normal. I mentioned earlier in this chapter that the ligaments in the ankle provide stability and prevent too much movement at the ankle joint; when the ligaments are stretched because the force on the ankle is greater than they can withstand, the ligaments are considered sprained. This happens when you land on an uneven surface and your foot rolls in, or if you fall, or if you step off of a curb funny and land on the outside of your foot. Remember how I said in Chapter 2 that ligaments are filled with cells that provide information about the body's location in space? When you overstretch ligaments, the proprioception of the joint is altered, often leading to feelings of instability or an ankle that feels "different" (Ritter & Moore 2008).

A clear demonstration of the concepts we have discussed so far can be seen in rehabilitation protocols for ballet dancers. Because dancers rely on proprioception and kinesthetic awareness in their feet and ankles for their work, effective rehabilitation for ankle sprains is critical. One form of rehabilitation that's used to treat ankle sprains involves exercises using a balance board with a textured surface (Steinberg et al. 2019). The textured surface allows the dancers to notice their feet more than normal because of the novel input. As a result, they make the appropriate adjustments with different parts of the foot to accommodate the textured surface. This is similar to what happens when you use a rock mat (a mat with small, rock-shaped objects on it). The sensory feedback from the mat on parts of the foot you don't usually use is strong. With practice, the foot learns to make small adjustments to allow the load across the foot to be dispersed more evenly and the input becomes less foreign, creating less discomfort.

The effects from ankle sprains can linger long after the initial injury, disrupting the ability to accurately feel both the position of the heel and its ability to make small movements. In one study, dancers with a history of ankle sprains were tested for their ability to determine the position of their heels. Before the intervention, they weren't as accurate at sensing heel position as their non-injured counterparts; after training on a textured surface balance board for 1 minute a day, every day for three weeks, their ability to determine heel position significantly improved. If students struggle with the above exercise of sensing foot position, using an exercise intervention that involves dynamically balancing on different surfaces may be an effective way to improve kinesthetic and proprioceptive awareness.

Asymmetry and laterality

Everyone is asymmetrical. I mentioned in Chapter 3 that the diaphragm looks like a lopsided mushroom, with the right side sitting higher in the ribcage than the left. There are also differences in the lungs; the right side of the lungs has three lobes and the left side only has two. The heart sits slightly to the left of the breastbone, and the liver, the largest organ in the body, is located in the right upper quadrant of the abdominal cavity, just below the diaphragm. Asymmetry, then, is a physiological occurrence.

Most people have a dominant hand they use for reaching, writing, and carrying things. This lateralization occurs at the level of the brain; it has been suggested this works well for efficiency and predictive control. When a movement can be done efficiently, with minimal neural noise, the end position tends to be more stable, which is beneficial for task success and completion (Sainburg 2014). Asymmetry is a neurological occurrence.

We live in a world where things are set up a certain way. Gas pedals are designed to be pushed with the right foot. Door handles usually turn clockwise; can openers turn clockwise and are designed to be held with the left hand, turned with the right hand. Asymmetry also occurs in the modern environment.

This works well for efficiency – I know if I want to open my front door, I need to turn the handle to the right. I don't need to ask myself which way to turn the handle every time I want to open the door. These natural tendencies become automatic, freeing up the brain for more important decisions like what's for dinner, or how you want to respond to

that uncomfortable work e-mail, or whether yoga pants are legitimate going-out apparel.

For people who move in varied ways regularly, the variety allows them to counteract the tendencies of anatomy, neurology, and convenience and still use both sides of their bodies. For people who move less often, asymmetries can become more habituated. Movement habits can become so entrenched, affecting body schema and motor schema, that the neuromuscular system "forgets" the wrist can rotate a different way or the foot can pronate and the ankle can evert. When it comes to motor control and movement, the old saying "use it or lose it" rings true.

In the foot-sensing exercise above, your feet may have felt really even, but when you looked down, perhaps your right foot was slightly behind the left foot or maybe the toes were turned a little bit to the right. When this happens, your *perception* of what was happening and what was actually happening didn't match. Even feet are by no means the Holy Grail and, for some people, may not even be a good idea because of the positions of their bones or a previous injury. The goal isn't to force the feet into parallel, but to practice having the ability to accurately gauge where the feet are in relation to each other to create a strong, clear foundation for balance and movement.

The position of the foot affects the shin, which affects the knee, which affects the femur, which affects the hip joint. Or maybe the hip joint affects the femur, which affects the knee, which affects the shin, which affects the foot? Regardless of which scenario is right, it's safe to say when you change the foot position, you are changing the position of the bones above the foot. The human body is predictable like that – it's all connected, so improving awareness and the use of the feet can sometimes create more freedom in the way the lower extremities move and interact with the environment.

Exercise
Lifting four toes

Come into a seated position with your bare feet on the ground or a standing position with your bare feet on the ground. Make sure you can look at your feet so you can see what's happening at the toes.

Press the big toe of the right foot into the ground and lift the other four toes up. Lower them down. Repeat four times and switch sides, performing the same movement on the left foot (Figure 5.1).

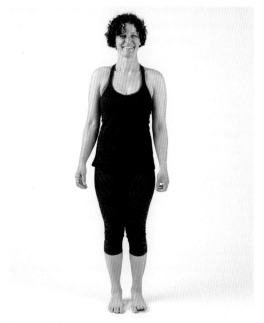

Figure 5.1

Though this seems like a simple isolation exercise, it can offer a number of clues about how a person uses their feet. Below are things to look for and some cueing suggestions to see if offering alternative options changes the student's strategy. The list is by no means exhaustive, and you may find yourself adding things you commonly see as you go through it.

Things to consider and observe

Does the person roll to the inside of the foot in order to keep the toes down? If yes, can they perform the same movement without rolling to the inside of the foot?

Do the toes scrunch or change shape when the person lifts them up? If yes, can they do it without them scrunching up?

Are the fingers or hands doing the motion at the same time that your toes do it? Can they do it without using the fingers and the hands?

Are they clenching their jaw or holding their breath? See if they can perform the movement while breathing and staying loose through the jaw area.

Is one foot harder than the other? If yes, take note of which side is easier.

The toes can move both in isolation and in a way that's integrated with the foot, just like the fingers can work independently and with the hand. One way to improve the body schema is to learn how to move body parts in isolation. The feet provide so much information to the neuromuscular system that having a clear sense of them, including the toes, makes the world feel safer. They are the body's connection with the physical environment most of the time. Plus, learning how to move the toes independently is an interesting party trick that will perplex other guests and make you a hit with your nephews.

What if your student simply can't do it, no matter how hard they scrunch their forehead and focus intently? What if the toes refuse to move and your student feels frustrated, completely disconnected from how to move the toes?

With practice, it will come, and the fun thing about the toes is it usually comes quickly. Performing any new movement or trying to isolate an area that hasn't been used in a while (or ever) takes a moment. Remember the phases of learning discussed in Chapter 4? Learning how to move the toes in the cognitive phase requires focused attention as the neuromuscular system spends time trying to figure out how many impulses to send to the area so that the movement can take place. Helping the neuromuscular system "figure out" the movement by pressing the big toe down with the hand, allowing the other toes to lift, or moving the toes up with the hand can teach the neuromuscular system how to create the action. Once the movement is understood cognitively, the associative stage of learning occurs, where the action of the toes lifting happens most of the time while the big toe stays down. The muscles of the toes are getting stronger during this phase and the neuromuscular system has figured out which motor units are required to perform the action. Eventually, the movement becomes fluid and can be done with a mere thought, placing the student in the autonomous phase of learning how to lift the toes.

Neuromuscular adaptations are the reasons people feel so much stronger four to six weeks after beginning a new exercise program. The muscles aren't physically stronger, but the neuromuscular system is learning how to perform the new task that's being asked of it, which is why understanding the phases of learning is helpful. At the end of the day, when you ask someone to perform a new movement or skill, you are asking the student to learn something new, whether it's lifting the toes, squatting a different way, or placing their body weight on their hands. The muscles and bones do adapt to the demands over time, becoming physiologically stronger to withstand the loads that are repeatedly being placed on the musculoskeletal system, but it is brain training first, muscle and bone training second (Bandy et al. 1990).

Exercise variation: the big toe

You can also perform the same exercise above while lifting just the big toe, while the other toes remain on the ground. Just like the toe-lifting exercise, asking people to lift the big toe can reveal how people use the foot to interact with the ground.

Things to consider and observe

- Does the big toe lift straight up or does it veer in (or out)?
- Do the other four toes scrunch or contract when the big toe lifts?
- Do the other four toes flatten when the big toe lifts?
- Does the big toe not lift off the ground at all?

If the big toe has difficulty lifting straight up, providing tactile feedback or an externally based cue can be beneficial. Placing a yoga block next to the big toe and keeping the big toe in contact with the block while trying to lift it is an example of using external feedback to perform the task.

The benefit of creating a scenario where the knowledge of successful task completion is clear is that the student knows right away whether they have been successful. If the toe doesn't stay against the block during the lift in the big toe task, the student knows they need to try a different strategy for the next attempt. This type of practice lends itself to skill learning and retention. The goal of an exercise and the feedback given should be to improve the student's understanding of the movement and the student's ability to replicate the skill and transfer the skill to other environments or conditions.

If the student is unable to lift the big toe without using the other toes, the student can use their hand to move the big toe manually. This is an example of concurrent feedback, or feedback that is given as the task is being performed. While concurrent feedback can be helpful in the moment and lead to immediate improvements, it does not appear to be beneficial for long-term retention. Augmented feedback, or feedback given after the task is performed, seems to be more effective for learning (Muratori et al. 2013). This doesn't mean not to use concurrent feedback; however, use it sparingly to build confidence and then use other forms of feedback to reinforce learning.

For the student attempting to keep their big toe against the block while lifting it, an example of augmented feedback would be the teacher assisting the student in understanding how they could perform the task more effectively. For instance, the teacher could suggest the student actively press the big toe into the block before attempting to lift the big toe, or the teacher could direct the student's attention to actively move the big toe away from the other toes as they try to lift the toe. Interestingly, research suggests less feedback is more effective for skill learning; as movement teachers, it can be tempting to offer suggestions after every attempt about how the skill could be performed more efficiently, but that may hinder the student's learning and their ability to transfer skills to other areas.

Another effective teaching tool is asking the student to visualize the task you are asking them to perform. For instance, asking the student to imagine the big toe is lifting straight up while the other toes stay down may be beneficial in helping the student understand how to perform the movement. When you imagine a motor task, the brain prepares to actually do the movement, so motor units are fired off, prepping the muscles for action (Bernardi et al. 2013). Visualizing can be a useful tool for improving the mind–body connection, filling in gaps in the body schema, and learning how to perform a wide variety of motor tasks, from lifting the big toe to walking up the stairs without pain to vaulting over a high wall smoothly.

When you walk, the foot pushes off of the ground. The heel lifts off of the ground, which means the toes extend. The big toe provides a platform for pushing. The only way the big toe can generate force is if it has the ability to extend, which gives it more leverage for pushing down.

When bunions are present, the big toe leans in toward the other toes, creating a bump on the outside of the big toe. The big toe may lose range of motion and strength, reducing its ability to act as a lever (InformedHealth.org 2018). The body and brain will work together to figure out another way to maintain balance and propel the body forward. Depending on the severity of the bunion, improving big toe mobility and strength in different positions may restore big toe function.

Exercise

Foot awareness using a towel

Come into a standing position. Take a moment to observe the weight of your feet against the floor. Which parts of the feet are heavy against the floor? Which parts are light? Is there more weight on the inside of the foot or the outside? What happens in the heel?

Roll up a small towel lengthwise, so it's not too thick, and it's wide enough that you can place

it underneath the ball of the foot. Stand up and place the rolled towel underneath the ball of the right foot. Make sure the right heel remains in contact with the floor.

Begin pressing the ball of the big toe joint into the towel. Feel how the pressure on the towel increases when you press the ball of the big toe into the towel. Hold for a moment or two and then relax. Repeat four times.

Now, press the ball of the little toe side of the foot into the towel. Hold for a couple of seconds and relax. Repeat four times.

Do the same thing with the ball of the second toe, fourth toe, and middle toe (Figure 5.2).

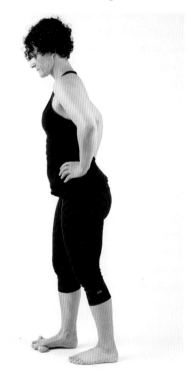

Figure 5.2

After you have finished, take the foot off the towel and pause for a moment. Feel the two feet against the floor. Do your feet feel different?

Repeat with the left foot. Once you have finished, observe the sensation of the feet. How do they feel? Can you feel different parts of your feet in contact with the ground?

Things to consider and observe

- Which areas are easiest to press down?

- Which are harder?

- Is the movement isolated at the forefoot, or is there a lot of movement in the ankle and knee?

- Is there a visible change in the student's connection with the ground after performing the exercise?

The towel acts as both proprioceptive feedback and as an external focus of attention. Because the towel feels different than the floor, the sensory receptors in the foot send afferent feedback to the brain about the texture and density of the towel. This increase in afferent information makes it easier for the student to feel the different parts of the foot pressing into the towel. You can do a similar exercise with the towel under the heel. If you don't have a towel, find an object that's slightly higher than the ground and a slightly different density. One of the easiest ways to improve connection with a specific body part is to place the body part in an environment where there is novel feedback. One of the strengths of the afferent nervous system is its ability to detect subtle changes; developing exercises that take advantage of the sensitivity of the afferent nervous system can assist with learning.

Developing kinesthetic awareness of the forefoot, the portion of the foot where the balls of the foot are located, can assist with balance. If someone primarily balances on the outside edge of the front of the foot will that feel more or less stable than balancing on the entire forefoot and the center of the heel?

Less stable, right? Helping people create a stable base to balance on by improving awareness through the foot increases confidence and makes it easier to integrate the foot into movement. One way to envision the balance points on the foot is to imagine it's shaped like a triangle, comprised of lines connecting the big toe ball of the foot to the pinkie toe ball of the foot to the center of the heel.

Exercise
Seated forefoot awareness

Come into a seated position, with the feet flat on the floor. Interlock your fingers, bend your torso down, and place your hands directly below the right knee cap. Your hands are there to make sure the knee doesn't move from side to side.

Keeping the right foot in contact with the floor, roll the pressure from the big toe side of the foot to the pinkie toe side of the foot and back to the big toe part of the foot. It's like you are waving the pressure across the foot, slowly and thoughtfully. Perform six to eight passes both ways and switch sides (exercise adapted from Elphinston 2013) (Figure 5.3).

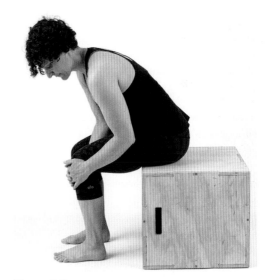

Figure 5.3

Things to consider and observe

Do you feel how your arch changes shape as you wave the pressure? At what point is the arch closest to the ground? When is it farther away from the ground?

- Does your knee stay still, or do you feel it wanting to move?

Chapter 5

- Can you feel the bone beneath your hands (the tibia), responding to the movement?

- Is it easier to wave one way versus another?

- Is it easier to do with one of your feet? If so, what makes it hard on the hard side?

You probably noticed that even though this exercise is performed seated and in a slightly different way, it is similar to the exercise with the towel. This is because one of the best ways to teach someone a skill is to have them perform similar actions, many different ways. Skill acquisition is characterized by consistency and flexibility. Flexibility can be thought of as the ability to adapt the skill appropriately for the environment. Asking someone to perform supination and pronation with a flexed knee is different than having the person do it with an extended knee, just like drawing attention to keeping the knee still is different than focusing attention on pressing different parts of the foot into a towel (Januario et al. 2016). If the goal is for the student to be able to perform movement and skills autonomously, teaching the same concept in a variety of ways improves skill flexibility and the ability to transfer the skill to multiple contexts.

Understanding how the foot affects tibial rotation can help the student create a much clearer image of the lower extremity. When the foot flattens, moving into pronation, the tibia, otherwise known as the shin bone, responds to the movement by internally rotating. When the arch lifts away from the floor, moving into supination, the tibia externally rotates. The femur, or long thigh bone, will also respond by internally rotating when the tibia internally rotates or externally rotating when the tibia externally rotates. The subtle movement that happens at the arch every time you walk causes a chain reaction throughout the leg (Hintermann & Nigg 1998; Rodrigues et al. 2015). This responsiveness is what enables you to change directions quickly without placing large amounts of stress on the knee and also creates the opportunity to get into interesting positions when you are playing on the playground.

Sometimes, bones don't coordinate smoothly, or one bone moves more than another, which is what often

happens when a joint lacks sufficient range of motion needed for the task. Joint range of motion can be thought of as the amount of movement available at a joint (Konin & Jessee 2012). Range of motion can be affected by a number of factors, including genetics, trauma, and disuse.

Having a student perform subtle movements and asking the student to observe how they respond connects them with which movements they do easily and which are more challenging or are difficult to feel. It also creates the opportunity to detect small changes in position, which is a useful way to improve your kinesthetic awareness (Rosker & Sarabon 2010). If a student struggles with a specific range of motion, moving slowly and gently begins to reestablish range of motion in the joint and coordinate the movements in a more fluid, non-threatening way. The foot, as important as it is, doesn't make big, sweeping movements like the thigh or shoulder. Paying attention to the subtlety of the feet and learning to control foot movement facilitates efficiency and balance in more dynamic, integrated skills.

Movement at the heel, or rearfoot, is partially dependent on whether the forefoot can efficiently move into abduction and adduction. These movements occur in the frontal plane and are important for allowing supination and pronation, the triplanar movements of the foot required for efficient walking I have referenced throughout the chapter.

The ankle joint can plantar flex and dorsiflex the foot. While it appears these movements occur in the sagittal plane, the complexity of the foot and ankle joint actually means all movement at the foot and ankle happens in a multi-planar way. When the foot is fixed, plantar flexion is comprised of tibial external rotation and foot supination; closed-chain dorsiflexion is comprised of tibial internal rotation and foot pronation (Chan & Rudins 1994).

The ankle can also plantar flex and dorsiflex in an open-chain environment, with the foot off of the ground. Plantar flexion happens when toes move away from the body and the heel moves toward the body. Dorsiflexion occurs when the toes move toward the body and the heel moves away from the body. These movements happen at the ankle joint and can be done without moving the toes. If the toes are involved in plantar flexion and dorsiflexion, the movement is then coupled with movement at the toe joints.

Movement at the ankle joint can manipulate the foot to move in a variety of ways, abducting and adducting the foot, internally and externally rotating the foot, and, as discussed above, plantar flexing and dorsiflexing the foot. It is possible to gain control of the ankle and move the foot without moving the toes; it's also possible to move the foot without moving the knee, isolating movement purely at the ankle joint.

When people struggle with isolating movement at the ankle joint, efficiency in the lower extremity is compromised. Re-establishing the ability to move the ankle in isolation can improve coordination and efficiency of the entire leg, improving load dispersal and coordination throughout the entire kinetic chain.

Exercise

Open-chain plantar flexion and dorsiflexion with feedback

Come into a seated position. Extend your right leg straight out in front of you, so your right heel is on the floor and your toes point straight up toward the ceiling.

Keeping the leg straight, slide the heel toward you, so the toes move away from you. Slide the heel away from you, so the toes move toward you. Repeat six times and then switch sides (Figures 5.4 and 5.5).

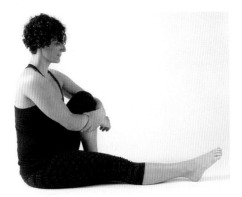

Figure 5.4

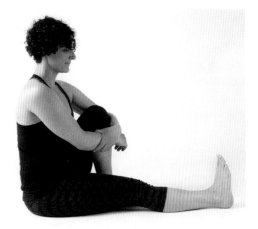

Figure 5.5

Things to consider and observe

- Can you slide the heel without flexing or extending the toes, or do the toes move when you slide the heel?

- Does the heel slide in a straight line?

- Is it difficult to keep the knee straight as you perform the movement?

After performing the movement seated, it can be interesting to perform the same action standing, observing whether the weight rolls to the outside or the inside of the foot as the heel moves away from the ground and back toward the ground. Because there is very little load in the seated variation of the exercise, it's often easier for people to "get" how to isolate and coordinate the movement. In the standing variation, there is a decreased sense of safety because of the increased balance demands and the increase in load. Another option is to face a wall and place the fingers lightly on the wall as the student lifts and lowers the heels. This increases the sense of safety and allows the student to focus their attention on performing the exercise with weight evenly distributed across the ball of the foot and/or observe whether there is a tendency to roll to the outside or inside of the foot while performing the action.

If the student struggles to place weight on the big toe side of the foot when the heel lifts off the ground, what does that tell you about how the student uses their foot?

Chapter 5

Remember earlier when I said plantar flexion couples with supination and tibial external rotation? More than likely, the student struggles with foot supination if they are rolling away from the big toe side of the foot. What else might you look for in this example? You may want to check how the student uses their big toe and if the student is able to keep the big toe actively pressing into the ground during supination. Finally, checking whether the student is able to control tibial internal and external rotation in closed chain will give you the information needed to know where to focus attention and direct cueing.

Ankle eversion and inversion – review

Earlier, I had you set a timer and practice performing eversion and inversion in different positions, based on your understanding of the movement. To recap, ankle eversion happens when the inside of the heel comes closer to the ground and ankle inversion happens when the outside of the heel comes closer to the ground. During quiet standing, it is efficient from both a neuromuscular and biomechanical standpoint to stand in a position where the center of the heel is in contact with the floor and the heel is neither inverted nor everted.

Different activities and terrains require varying degrees of ankle mobility. Teaching students how to gradually load the inside and outside of the feet strengthens the tissues; it also increases proprioceptive and kinesthetic awareness of the area and builds confidence in the ankle joint and its ability to tolerate different positions.

Exercise
Ankle mobility – closed-chain plantar flexion and dorsiflexion

Come into a standing position. Without looking down, notice where the weight is in your heels. Is it in the center of the heels or on the inside or the outside of the heels? Or maybe it's different between the feet?

Look down at your heels and check their position. You may have to look behind you to actually see what's happening. Is what's happening in your heels what you thought was happening?

Lift the heels off the ground, balancing your weight on your forefoot. If this feels scary or throws your balance off, lift just one heel a few times and then do the other (Figure 5.6).

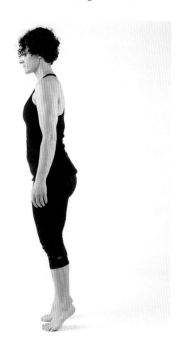

Figure 5.6

Try lifting the forefoot off the ground a few times, coming onto your heels. See how that feels. Is it easier or harder than lifting the heels of the feet up?

Stand quietly and feel your heels against the floor. Do they feel different?

Things to consider and observe

- Is it plantar flex (lift the heels) to dorsiflex the feet in standing?

- Do the movements look fluid and controlled, or choppy and slightly uncoordinated?

- Can the student perform the movements without looking at their feet?

- Does the weight disperse evenly across the ball of the foot during plantar flexion or does the weight roll to the inside (or outside) of the ball of the foot?

- What happens when the student dorsiflexes? Does the weight move toward the inside or the outside of the heel when the forefoot lifts?

Lifting different parts of the feet off of the ground reinforces the many ways the feet can move. It establishes a clear image of the heels and where they are in relation to the ground. A sense of safety increases when movements are performed in a controlled manner and in a situation where there is enough feedback to feel specific areas of the body. Giving students time to process their experience by asking questions that require reflection improves learning and transfer of skills. As you have learned throughout this chapter, the feet are complex; creating opportunities for students to learn how they function and the way the rest of the body responds to their movements is an interesting way to enhance mindful movement and coordination.

Chapter 5

Case study: ankle sprain

I worked with a woman for a few months who had sprained her ankle many years ago. The ankle never fully recovered, and she never quite trusted it to support her. She had given up shoes with a heel, even a small one, and was pretty sure she was destined to be careful walking on uneven surfaces for the rest of her life.

During one of our first sessions together, I had her take her shoes off. I worked with her on feeling the feet against the floor and balancing on one leg. I had her do movements similar to what I described above, and challenged her to walk on uneven surfaces. When our time together ended, she thanked me profusely for giving her back the ability to use her ankle. She could wear shoes with a small heel and no longer felt like it was going to give out on her when she walked on trails. She had more stability and strength in her ankle than she had had in years, and for that she was grateful.

Over the course of this chapter, I have discussed how the foot works in gait, and why balance training is important for ankle sprains. I have provided examples of exercises that can be used to improve awareness, but these are just examples. Once you understand the basic concepts of how movement is sensed and performed, you can create exercises that are appropriate for the student's individualized situation.

When you are working with someone with foot and ankle injuries, it's important to challenge balance gradually, in a way that doesn't feel threatening, so the student can focus on the subtle aspects of movement in the foot and ankle. Remember, proprioception improves when you use your joints; the more control, mobility, and strength someone has in their feet, the better their proprioception will be, impacting balance and coordination. In the case study above, my client's proprioception was altered. This isn't uncommon in injuries like ankle sprains because ligaments have been stretched. This creates feelings of instability that can last long after everything is healed (Tropp 2002). However, the feelings of instability don't have to be permanent. With the appropriate movement intervention, the perception of the ankle can change, improving confidence and strength.

References

Bandy WD, Lovelace-Chandler V, and McKitrick-Bandy B (1990) Adaptation of skeletal muscle to resistance training. Journal of Orthopaedic & Sport Physical Therapy 12 (6) 248–255.

Bernardi NF, De Buglio MD, Trimarchi PD, Chielli A, and Bricolo E (2013) Mental practice promotes motor anticipation: Evidence from skilled music performance. Frontiers in Human Neuroscience 7 451.

Brockett CL and Chapman GJ (2016) Biomechanics of the ankle. Orthopaedics & Trauma 30 (3) 232–238.

Chan CW and Rudins A (1994) Foot biomechanics during walking and running. Mayo Clinic Proceedings 69 (5) 448–461.

Chou S-W, Cheng H-Y.K, Chen J-H, Ju Y-Y, Lin Y-C, and Wong M-K A (2009) The role of the great toe in balance performance. Journal of Orthopaedic Research 27 (4) 549–554.

Elphinston J (2013) Stability, sport and performance movement: Practical biomechanics and systematic training for movement efficacy and injury prevention. Chichester, UK: Lotus Publishing.

Han BI, Song HS, and Kim JS (2011) Vestibular rehabilitation therapy: Review of indications, mechanisms, and key exercises. Journal of Clinical Neurology 7 (4) 184–196.

Han J, Anson J, Waddington G, Adams R, and Liu Y (2015) The role of ankle proprioception for balance control in relation to sport performance and injury. Biomed Research International. doi: 10.1155/2015/842804.

Highstein SM (2004) Anatomy and physiology of the central and peripheral vestibular system: Overview, in Highstein SM, Fay RR, and Popper AN (eds) The vestibular system. Springer handbook of auditory research, vol. 19. New York, NY: Springer.

Hintermann B and Nigg BM (1998) Pronation in runners. Implications for injuries. Sports Medicine 26 (3) 169–176.

Hughes J, Clark P, and Klenerman L (1990) The importance of the toes in walking. Journal of Bone and Joint Surgery 72 (2) 245–251.

InformedHealth.org [Electronic] (2006) Cologne, Germany: Institute for Quality and Efficiency in Health Care (IQWiG) Bunions: Overview. June 28, 2018. Available: https://www.ncbi.nlm.nih.gov/books/NBK513134/.

Januario MS, Ugrinowitsch H, Lage GM, Viera M, and Benda RN (2016) Gradual increment on practice variability: Effects on structure learning and skill parametrization. Revista Brasileira de Educação Física e Esporte [Brazilian Journal of Physical Education and Sport] 30 (3) 781–791 .

Konin JG and Jessee B (2012) Range of motion and flexibility, in Andrews J, Harrelson G, and Wilk K (eds) Physical rehabilitation of the injured athlete, 4th edn. London, UK: Elsevier.

Lang J (2016) Small teachings: Everyday lessons from the science of learning. San Francisco, CA: Jossey-Bass.

Muratori LM, Lamberg EM, Quinn L, and Duff SV (2013) Applying principles of motor learning and control to upper extremity rehabilitation. Journal of Hand Therapy 26 (2) 94–103.

Ridola CG, Cappello F, Marciano V, Francavilla C, Montalbano A, Farina-Lipari E, and Palma A (2007) The synovial joints of the human foot. Italian Journal of Anatomy and Embryology 112 (2) 61–81.

Ritter S and Moore M (2008) The relationship between lateral ankle sprain and ankle tendinitis in ballet dancers. Journal of Dance Medicine & Science 12 (1) 23–31.

Rockar PJ (1995) The subtalar joint: Anatomy and joint motion. Foot/Ankle Therapy & Research 21 (6) 361–372.

Rodrigues P, Chang R, TenBroek T, van Emmerik R, and Hamill J (2015) Evaluating the coupling between foot pronation and tibial internal rotation continuously using vector coding. Journal of Applied Biomechanics 31 (2) 88–94.

Rosker J and Sarabon N (2010) Kinaesthesia and methods for its assessment. Sports Science Review 5–6 (19) 165–208.

Sainburg RL (2014) Convergent models of handedness and brain lateralization. Frontiers in Psychology 5 1,092.

Steinberg N, Adams R, Tirosh O, Karin J, and Waddington G (2019) Effects of textured balance board training in adolescent ballet dancers with ankle pathology. Journal of Sports Rehabilitation 28 (6) 584–592.

Tropp H (2002) Commentary: Functional ankle instability revisited. Journal of Athletic Training 37 (4) 512–515.

van Deursen RW and Simoneau GG (1999) Foot and ankle sensory neuropathy, proprioception, and postural stability. Journal of Orthopedic Sport Physical Therapy 29 (12) 718–726.

Wright WG, Ivanenko YP, and Gurfinkel VS (2012) Foot anatomy specialization for postural sensation and control. Journal of Neurophysiology 107 (5) 1,513–1,521.

Case study

I have a client who began seeing me shortly after the birth of her daughter. She had been on bed rest during a portion of her pregnancy and had lost strength. She began experiencing persistent neck pain that became chronic and was affecting her ability to sleep and function. She was under the care of a massage therapist and a chiropractor, but she wanted to gain confidence in her ability to move without pain.

As I watched her move in our first session, I noticed she was struggling with using her feet for balance. Her eyes looked habitually toward the floor, to get the information she was lacking from her proprioceptive system. Her torso moved in a way that appeared unstable, responding to the lack of stability she felt in the feet and ankles.

I slowly began improving kinesthetic awareness of the feet and ankles through mobility and using foot-awareness exercises like the ones described in Chapter 5. I gave her opportunities to practice balancing in a safe environment, and I taught her how to feel her feet, rather than rely on her eyes. We also worked on basic strength exercises to re-establish a foundation for stability.

Her pain would disappear during our sessions, and as she became stronger and had a deeper sense of stability, the pain would be gone for longer and longer periods of time, until eventually it was gone completely.

Her lack of inactivity during bed rest resulted in the visual and vestibular systems becoming her main sources for maintaining balance. Because she had lost strength, her torso moved a lot when she was on one leg, acting like an extension of her ankle to keep her upright. Her head was like the top of a sail in the wind – there was a lot of movement below it, and the neck was working really hard to keep everything going in the right direction.

After we had been training together for about a year, she had her husband come in to see me for a consult. He looked at me and said, "Since she's been working with you, her confidence level has grown. It's impacted her in a positive way, both professionally and personally. I'm not sure what you guys do, and she always says you are training her for the circus, but whatever it is, it's working." Improving her confidence in her body's ability to support her led to more confidence in other areas of her life.

In the previous chapters, we spent a lot of time discussing the foundations of movement. While we touched upon balance in Chapter 5 when we explored the feet, this chapter will tie many of the concepts we have already discussed together through understanding how balance can relate to the mind and the body, and the influences the mind and the body can have on each other.

Emotional balance, like physical balance, is determined by a variety of factors. To be emotionally balanced means you are able to feel a full spectrum of emotions while returning to a baseline that is fairly neutral. You can honestly assess how you feel without reacting, and while you can be flexible with how you are feeling based on the situation, you can recognize your emotions for what they are (Grecucci et al. 2015).

Physical balance is the ability to respond to perturbations, or outside forces, which alter your position. Balance happens when you recover from the perturbation and return to the original, stable position.

Mindfulness (see Chapter 4) is an effective way to establish emotional balance, reduce anxiety (Goldin & Gross 2010), and decrease the occurrence of depression (Bondolfi et al. 2010). Having emotional balance positively impacts relationships, daily function, and the ability to deal with stress; practicing mindfulness, specifically open monitoring and focused attention, disrupts the activity in the brain associated with mind-wandering. Another name for this area is the default mode network (Fujino et al. 2018).

continued

Chapter 6

Case study *continued*

Practicing mindfulness also improves cognitive performance, well-being, and daily happiness.

Emotions such as anger, fear, or stress cause physiological changes to occur. Heart rate increases and respiration changes, becoming slightly quickened and shallower. The pupils dilate, and muscles tense as sympathetic nervous system activity is increased (McCorry 2007). The chemicals associated with the sympathetic nervous system, specifically norepinephrine, are the same chemicals that are released during exercise. Exercise, then, can be thought of as a form of graded exposure therapy for people who associate the interoceptive sensations of increased heart rate and respiration rate with feelings of stress or panic. Becoming habituated to the sensations related to exercise is one of the reasons researchers speculate aerobic exercise may be an effective treatment for people experiencing chronic anxiety (Stonerock et al. 2015).

When feelings of anger or fear pass, the physiological makeup changes again. Sympathetic nervous system activity decreases and parasympathetic nervous system activity increases, creating an emotional balance. If those feelings don't pass, and the anger, anxiety, or stress become chronic, your sense of emotional strength and well-being is impacted, affecting your behavior and function throughout the day.

Physical balance works in a similar way. Pretend you are walking across the street and you don't see a pothole directly under where your left foot is about to land. As your left foot lands in the pothole, you feel unsteady, as though you are about to fall, but you catch yourself and keep walking (after glancing around to make sure no one saw you). The pothole caused a perturbation; your response demonstrated good interplay between the proprioceptive and vestibular systems, resulting in your ability to remain upright (Purves et al. 2001; Proske & Gandevia 2012). The vestibular system works with the

visual system to maintain gaze stability; gaze stability recovery is the first part of the balance recovery to occur, followed by postural stability recovery. Postural stability recovery is dependent on sensory information from the visual, vestibular, and somatosensory system; somatosensory information is largely reliant on the proprioceptive system (Han et al. 2011).

If the small deviation in the street was enough to knock you over and caused you to fall, the perturbation would have been greater than your proprioceptive, vestibular, and visual systems could handle. You would have been unable to recover your postural stability.

Having physical balance creates a sense of confidence during everyday activities. It reduces the fear associated with things like walking across a bridge or walking across a surface that's a little uneven. Just like with emotional balance, balance requires the flexibility to respond to perturbations; it also requires a sense of stability, of knowing what it means to feel centered.

Many of our traditional daily activities don't challenge the balance systems in a significant way. Balance becomes something that's ignored, and it isn't until you wake up one day realizing you have to sit down to put on your undergarments that you realize you've lost something. (I can't count how many clients come in after working with me for two to three months ecstatic that they can stand to put on their underpants in the morning. They whisper it, giddy, not wanting anyone else to hear.)

The importance of balance isn't confined to getting dressed. Poor balance is correlated with anxiety in adults (Rahimi & Abadi 2012) and anxiety and low self-esteem in children and the elderly (Bart et al. 2009; Carmeli 2015). In fact, anxiety and vestibular disorders appear to go hand in hand, suggesting that anxiety can be symptomatic of underlying health problems. Difficulty balancing

continued

Case study *continued*

and anxiety can lead to individuals avoiding social interactions and reducing their participation in daily activities. This decreases feelings of strength and autonomy and increases feelings of isolation.

Researchers have examined the correlation between anxiety and balance in mice by breeding mice to have the gene that results in balance deficits. Mice either lived in a cage that was filled with interesting balance challenges like balance beams and things to climb on and hang from or they spent their days in a cage that lacked physical obstacles. Balance improved and anxiety decreased in the mice that lived in the balance-enriched environment while the mice in the control group developed high levels of anxiety (Shefer et al. 2015).

Obviously, what happens in mice can't be extrapolated to the human experience; however, incorporating balance training for individuals with anxiety symptoms may be beneficial for reducing fear associated with falling and instability. While it's impossible to know whether the anxiety comes before the loss of balance or the loss of balance causes anxiety, it appears they often co-exist. The great news is, as evidenced by the mice, it's entirely possible to improve balance and reduce feelings of anxiety. Even if you are working with someone who isn't an anxious person, incorporating balance work is still beneficial for activities of everyday life, improving confidence and the sense of capability. Spending even a couple of minutes challenging balance daily is enough to have long-term benefits.

Exercise
Moving the head in space

Come into a standing position. Take a moment to feel how your feet are pressing into the floor and where you feel most of the weight. Is it in the front of your feet or in your heels? Is it on the left foot or the right foot?

Now, move your eyes to the left and let your head go, too. It's like there is an object to the left of you and you are trying to reach it with your head. Let your head and your eyes return to center. Repeat this three or four times and then do the same on the right (Figure 6.1).

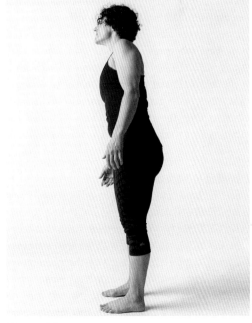

Figure 6.1

Imagine there is an object in front of you. Let your eyes and your head begin reaching toward it. Return the head and the eyes back to the starting position. Repeat this three or four times. Now, imagine there is an object up on the ceiling and behind you that you want to reach. Look up and behind you for the object and reach your head toward the object. Return the head and the eyes back to center. Repeat this three or four times and come back to the original standing position.

How does the weight feel in your feet now? Has anything changed?

Before you move on, set a timer for 2 minutes. Try reaching from your head in a variety of positions. How does it feel? Are any of the positions more challenging than others?

After the timer goes off, notice your head. Does it feel light? Heavy? How does your neck feel?

Reaching a body part toward something is an example of using an external stimulus to encourage a specific behavior. Reaching feels different than contracting, which feels different than stretching, which feels different than pushing … you get the idea. The goal of this specific exercise is to increase awareness of the head and eyes in various positions. As a result, I chose the words "reach toward" to encourage a relaxed movement that may or may not involve other body parts. I purposefully didn't specify whether to keep the rest of the body still because in dynamic balance work, the body is responsive, not rigid.

Because the eyes and head are instrumental for maintaining balance, it's important to utilize movements that use the head and the eyes in different positions. If you only think of balance training as standing on one leg, you aren't utilizing two-thirds of the systems that keep you upright. Practicing movements with the head and eyes creates a more complete integration of the neuromuscular system and begins to allow the student to practice gaze stability recovery in a situation that feels safe. During head-turning movements, the eyes move earlier (and faster) than the head. For the duration of the head movement, the eyes

remain fixed while the head continues to turn, creating stability (Dichgans et al. 1973; Diehl & Pidcoe 2006).

In life, balance is a dynamic activity. It can be thought of as alternating between phases of stress, recovery, and stability. The balance system is used every time you transition between static postures. Balance can be challenged a number of ways, including when the head turns quickly, there is an unexpected curb on the street, or something happens that requires you to quickly change position. Throw in an uneven surface that isn't uniform, and the balance system is required to rapidly and dynamically maintain postural stability. Another way to think of balance is as the ability to adapt to a variety of conditions and remain upright; movement training, then, should emphasize movement that occurs in different planes and on a variety of surfaces.

The planes of movement

I have mentioned the planes of movement periodically up until now, but I haven't defined them. From a biomechanical perspective, there are three planes of movement: sagittal, frontal, and transverse.

Sagittal movement occurs in a forward and back manner. When you raise your arm directly in front of you or directly behind you, that is movement in the sagittal plane. Sagittal plane movement is commonly associated with flexion and extension.

Frontal plane movement is movement that happens directly to the side of you. If we stick with our arm example, if I were to reach my arm directly out to the side of the body, that would be movement in the frontal plane. Frontal plane movement is associated with abduction and adduction.

Transverse plane movement occurs horizontally. If I reach my arm across the body, I am moving in the transverse plane. Transverse plane movement is rotational joint movement.

Each synovial joint has the ability to move in the sagittal, frontal, and transverse planes. Remember how in

Chapter 5 we talked about tibial internal rotation? That is a rotational movement of the tibia occurring in the transverse plane. When you extend the leg from the knee joint, that is movement at the sagittal plane, and when the right knee moves toward the left knee, that is adduction of the knee joint that is happening in the frontal plane. When you walk, movement occurs in the frontal, sagittal, and transverse plane at the knee joint, responding to the rotational actions of the foot and hip; to an outsider watching someone walk, the gross motor pattern appears to happen in the sagittal plane. It's only if you look more carefully that you see that walking, or any movement, is a three-dimensional experience of rotational movements occurring in all three planes (Stoelben et al. 2019).

In order for movement to be coordinated, when one area moves, another responds. This is what creates the ability to respond to a perturbation. In order to maintain postural stability for daily tasks, for instance, movement happens in the trunk while the head usually performs a countermovement relative to the trunk or torso to maintain a consistent head orientation (Peeters et al. 2018). The coordination of movements for daily activities is usually subtle because prior experience performing activities of daily living leads to motor control coordination and efficiency. Teaching students to be responsive to perturbations rather than stiff can improve motor control and enhance variability; however, a degree of joint mobility and general strength is required for students to feel safe during any kind of perturbation training.

Exercise
Changing the base of support

Come into a standing position. Lift your heels off of the floor so the weight is evenly distributed across the balls of the feet. Take three steps forward and three steps backward. Set the heels down as needed to maintain balance.

Once you are finished, lower your heels down and lift the front of your feet up, taking three steps forward and three steps backward.

Things to observe and ask

- Which condition felt less awkward?

- Do you prefer going forward or backward?

- Where did you look when your heels were off of the ground? What about when the front of your feet were off of the ground?

Limiting the amount of contact the feet have with the floor changes the amount of feedback the brain receives from all of the mechanoreceptors in the feet – there will be less, which means the visual and vestibular system will kick into high gear to maintain stability. It also decreases the base of support. Base of support is defined as the area beneath a person, including all of the contact points the person's body makes with the supporting surface. As I mentioned earlier, the heel provides stability and support for the lower extremity. Removing the heel (or front of the foot) from the ground significantly changes a person's base of support.

The other thing that changes when the heels lift away from the floor is a person's center of mass. The center of mass is the place in the body where the body's mass is equally distributed in all directions. It, too, is dependent on a variety of factors, including position of the limbs and gender. Generally speaking, the center of mass is a little bit lower than the belly button, just in front of the second sacral vertebrae. What happens to the center of mass when the heels lift away from the floor? It moves up because the torso moves up. It's still located in the same place, it's just that the position of the body has shifted. Do you think that it would be more or less difficult to balance with a center of mass that is suddenly higher?

Most people find it more challenging, and that's because of gravity. If you were to crouch down with your heels lifted, your center of mass would be lower to the ground and you would be more compact. You would feel more stable because you aren't resisting gravity as much. If you have ever done any contact improvisation or Acroyoga, you have experienced how when your partner changes shape, it changes how you have to support them to maintain a sense of stability. The body and its center of mass change with every position; altering foot contact with the floor is a simple way to practice changing center of mass in an environment where it's safe to observe tendencies.

You already know the ankles are an important source of proprioceptive information and that they play an important role in gait. You may also know that as you age, your risk for falling increases; research suggests that more than one-third of the population aged 65 or older will fall each year; the risk goes up if you have a history of falling (Al-Aama 2014). As you age, joints change. There is less water content in the cartilage, and synovial joint fluid and proteoglycans decrease, affecting joint mobility. Several studies have shown a 12–30% decrease in plantar flexion–dorsiflexion and inversion–eversion at the ankle joint in older adults. That's a big range, indicating other factors likely contribute to the decrease in ankle mobility, not just the physiological changes related to aging. Asking people to use the joint mobility they have by loading the joint in a variety of ways and coordinating the joint with the entire body during movement tasks is a way to maintain function and possibly reduce the age-related risk of falling (Menz 2015).

Practical application

Set a timer for 3 minutes. Make different positions with your body. Pause in each position and think about where the center of mass is located. How would someone most efficiently balance you in the position? Which positions create the easiest balance point? Which create the most challenging?

Once the feet are strong enough, you can alter foot position by using exercises like squatting variations, lunging variations, and walking variations. As long as new movements are introduced gradually and the joints are responsive and coordinating with one another, you as the practitioner are only limited by your creativity.

Exercise
Heel to toe walking

Make sure you have a clear space. Place your right heel directly in front of your left toes. Then place your left heel directly in front of your right toes, so you are walking forward heel to toe. Take about eight steps. Try the same thing going backward (Figure 6.2).

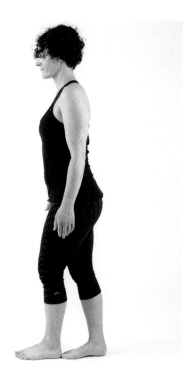

Figure 6.2

Things to observe and ask

- Where were the hands? Were they tensed or relaxed?
- Where did the eyes look?
- How much movement occurred in the torso?
- Are you breathing?

Walking heel to toe poses an interesting balance challenge for many people. In order to maintain a base of support, the front foot has to move into pronation as weight is transferred on to it. If someone has a habit of avoiding pronation, they either adapt with joints further up the kinetic chain, maintaining balance while avoiding pronation, or lose their balance. What way will someone fall if their habit is avoiding pronation on their right foot?

They would likely fall to the right. Avoiding pronation is often coupled with the inability to actively press the big toe into the ground, which means the weight in our hypothetical student would be mostly on the outside of the foot. Learning how to walk heel to toe in a situation where there is no imminent threat gives the neuromuscular system a chance to figure out which options are available to perform the task without requiring much instruction from you, the teacher. If someone were unable to understand the movement required to complete the act of walking heel to toe successfully, what options do you have for helping the student "get" it?

You have two choices: you can either give the person feedback or you can have the student perform an awareness drill such as the listening foot exercise in Chapter 5 that teaches the foot actions that occur at the subtalar joint and have the person try the exercise again, hoping the skill transfers.

If you choose to give feedback, when would you give feedback so that it is most optimal for learning?

This gets tricky because augmented feedback, or feedback given from a teacher to a student to enhance skill performance, can either help or hinder learning, depending on when and how it is given (Magill 1994). The teacher has a choice: give feedback during the skill or give feedback after the student has finished walking heel to toe. Which is more effective?

The effectiveness of when the feedback is given depends on what type of cue you choose to give. Concurrent cues are cues that are given as the student is performing the desired skill. If you give a concurrent intrinsic cue, or a cue that is directed toward how the student is achieving the task, you will likely see an immediate improvement of the skill, but the ability of the student to replicate the skill successfully next week is low. If you give a concurrent extrinsic cue, the student may not perform the skill as well in the moment, but, next week, the likelihood of the student being able to perform the skill successfully is high (Wulf 2007).

For example, while the student was walking heel to toe, if you asked the student to focus on actively pressing the big toe side of the foot down, that would be an example of a concurrent intrinsic cue. If you asked the student to keep the inside of the foot in contact with the floor, that would be an example of an extrinsic cue. In the first example, the student is being asked to manipulate their foot in a way that achieves the desired result. In the second example, the student is being asked to focus on feeling the floor. Both cues achieve the same thing, but they are processed differently by the student.

On the other hand, if feedback were given immediately after the skill or was delayed and given some time before the next balancing attempt, either an intrinsic or extrinsic cue would likely have been retained making the next attempt successful.

Ultimately, when you give the cue and which type of cue you give is determined by the goal behind the exercise. Do you want your student to perform the skill well right now? Or do you want the student to perform the skill well in the future?

Another way to make the skill more accessible is to have the student extend their arms out to the sides while walking heel to toe. The arms act as levers, making it easier to feel where the balance point is located. Imagine the approximate location of the center of mass (slightly below the belly button and in front of the second sacral vertebrae). When the arms are extended out to the sides, if you were to draw a line from the hands to the center of mass, it would resemble a triangle, with the center of mass acting as balancing point for the two sides. Since the base of support, or area where the feet connect to the ground, is narrow, holding the arms out to the side makes the balance point of the body more obvious, allowing the neuromuscular system to self-organize and maintain postural stability.

You could also give the student a weighted object to hold, such as a sandbag or medicine ball, creating a constraint in the upper body. A constraint is defined as any task, environmental, or individual-related factor that influences the outcome of an observed motor pattern. The task constraint imposed by the weight limits the degrees of freedom available in the upper extremity and requires the student to adapt to the demands of the environment, specifically the weight and the balance task (Davids et al. 2006). The degrees of freedom are the amount of options the student has available for performing the task of walking heel to toe. The number of degrees of freedom available depends on how much mobility is available at each joint; the addition of the weight prevents movement in the arms. Reducing the degrees of freedom available at a specific joint gives the nervous system fewer options for task performance (Li 2006). Additionally, if you remember from Chapter 2 that one way to improve proprioception is through force, the external weight requires the student to contract muscles in order to hold the weight, improving stability through improved proprioception.

Both holding the arms out to the side and holding a weight are examples of exercise progressions that provide intrinsic feedback. This means the student can feel whether or not the suggested change has made the exercise easier or more challenging and whether or not they are able to complete the task successfully. Changing the arm position or adding load will change the way the student uses their feet without you giving additional cueing.

Placing a student in a situation where they have to balance requires micro-adjustments in the torso as it responds to gravity. Sometimes, these adjustments are big and more obvious, especially if it's the first time the student has been exposed to a particular balance challenge. As the student moves from the cognitive phase of learning to the associative phase of learning, the adjustments become small, almost imperceptible to the observer.

A common strategy used when students are initially exposed to a new – and potentially threatening – situation is breath-holding. Breath-holding creates a temporary sense of stability in the torso, causing it to become rigid and preventing excess movement. If the neuromuscular system feels unstable, it will create stability however it can to remain upright and safe. Breath-holding can be thought of as a high threshold stability strategy, which means there are circumstances, such as lifting heavy loads, where it might be a good choice. During low-threshold activities such as walking heel to toe, breath holding is not only unnecessary, it will likely reduce the student's likelihood of success. A stiff spine is not a responsive spine; responsiveness optimizes the neuromuscular system's ability to recover and right itself.

Other common ways to reduce movement in the torso include pulling the belly button in toward the spine (abdominal hollowing) and consciously contracting the muscles in the torso (abdominal bracing) (Kim & Kim 2018). Here's the thing about consciously trying to contract the abdominals: unless you are recovering from a neurological event that affected your neuromuscular control, such as a stroke, your nervous system knows which muscles need to work to keep you stable without you consciously trying to alter anything (Mehta et al. 2017). This means that when you ask someone to contract the abdominals while performing a dynamic balance activity, it interferes with their body's natural stabilization strategy during a low-threshold activity, again making their spine less responsive and able to recover.

This doesn't mean you can't help someone become more connected to their center of mass while dynamically balancing, or that the student won't feel the sensation of abdominal work. If the student's tendency is to lean back, flaring their ribs away from their pelvis while they walk heel to toe, do you think this is going to be more or less stable than keeping the ribs in a more expiratory position, like we discussed in Chapter 3? When you lift the ribs away from the pelvis, you move the ribs away from the center of mass. This makes the body less stable. Think of it this way: is there more movement when you push the center of a slinky that has one side in contact with the ground and the coils resting on top of it or a slinky with one side resting on the ground and the other side pulled away from the bottom? In the second scenario, when I push the center of the spread-out slinky there will be more visible movement than if I push the center of the more compact slinky. While the ribs and the pelvis don't exactly resemble a slinky because of lumbar and thoracic curves, when the upper half of the torso is lifted away from the center of mass, it requires more work to recover from perturbations. Lowering the ribs connects the upper torso extremities to the center of mass, changing the balance point of the body to a more advantageous position, increasing stability. One way to create awareness of the rib cage area in a situation that may feel stressful is to ask the student to pause and notice the breath. If the exhale feels short, letting out a quiet sigh or long exhale and feeling how the ribs respond focuses the attention on something other than the challenging task and connects the student with the center of their body. You can also give the student a weighted object, like that suggested above, which usually places the ribs in a more expiratory position without extra cueing. Knowing which intervention is appropriate depends on what the student needs in the moment.

Try this: set a timer for 3 minutes. Practice a controlled fall to the floor using a variety of stabilization strategies, such as holding the breath, tightening the abs, breathing easily, and hollowing the belly. Which strategy allows you to create the most softness through your torso? If you've never tried practicing controlled falls, try to make your way easily to the ground instead, imagining you are loose, like a rag doll. Where do you hold access tension? Where

can you be more soft and responsive? Practicing falling makes the ground less scary and creates empathy for how your students feel when they are placed in new balance situations.

Exercise
Creating perturbations using the upper body

Come into a standing position. Notice the weight of your feet on the ground.

Set a timer for 1 minute. Begin reaching the right arm to different areas. Reach it in front of you, to the right, down and to the left, behind you … any way you can think of to reach the right arm, reach it. Let your eyes follow the right hand (Figures 6.3–6.5).

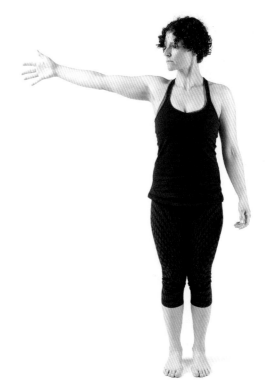

Figure 6.3

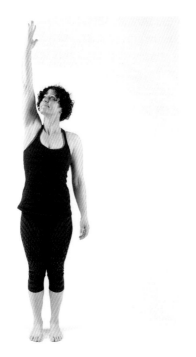

Figure 6.4

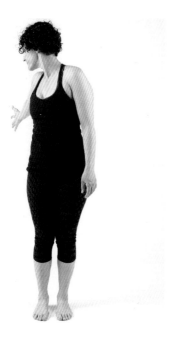

Figure 6.5

As you get comfortable with the act of reaching your arms, play with transferring the weight to your left foot, lifting your weight heel and hovering the right foot off the ground. Set the heel down as needed.

When the timer goes off, switch to the other side.

Things to observe and ask

- What does the spine do as the arms reach?

- How does the weight shift in the torso and stabilizing leg?

- Is one side easier than the other?

- Where do the eyes look?

When the arms move to different places, the spine will move more. It's the nature of how the body works: the upper extremity attaches to the torso by the shoulder blades, so creating movement in the arms creates movement in the spine. However, too much spinal movement will throw you off balance; dynamic balance is the constant quest for the sweet spot between stiffness and flexibility.

I have incorporated balance training into my work with clients for several years. During that time, I have noticed there is one thing that consistently improves people's ability to move with more control in the spine and that is gaining strength. Strength can be accomplished in many ways, but the basic rule of thumb for strength is when load causes stress to the musculoskeletal system, physiological adaptation takes place in the form of increased ability to withstand load in the muscles, tendons, ligaments, and bones. Load can be applied using gravity, such as with body weight exercises like pull-ups, ring work, or push-ups, or using an external implement such as a barbell, kettlebell, or even a rock. Regardless of which tool you choose, strength equates to force, which equates to better proprioception and, as a result, better balance.

One of the things I often do with my clients in order to give them time to process is to ask them questions about their experience with a skill or movement after it's over. I do this because self-reflection expedites the learning process by focusing attention and piquing curiosity. If I ask a question and the client is unsure, they focus their attention on the next set so they can answer my question.

There are two types of feedback that can be provided to improve motor learning: knowledge of performance and knowledge of results. Knowledge of performance is feedback that informs how an individual is performing a skill. How are they using their arms to walk heel to toe? Which part of the foot are they using? This form of feedback can be beneficial for establishing a mind–body connection and enhancing proficiency, particularly in the cognitive stages of learning.

Knowledge of results is feedback that is given regarding whether or not the skill was completed successfully. In the arm reaching example, if the student falls off balance and needs to place the entire foot back on the ground, the attempt was unsuccessful. This type of feedback requires less cueing from the coach and is effective for improving skill efficiency, particularly in the later stages of learning (Sunaryadi 2017).

Most teachers use both forms of feedback to enhance a student's performance. When you ask a student to reflect on their performance, they are providing knowledge of performance feedback with regards to how they performed the task using intrinsic feedback.

Again, it's important to know what your goals are as a teacher. If the goal is for the student to perform the skill in a consistent, efficient way, pay attention to how you cue matters. Too much instruction may result in the student being reliant on the instructor's feedback, hindering the student's ability to perform the movement on their own. Too little feedback doesn't create self-awareness around how the skill is being performed and pique curiosity about how it can be performed differently.

Walking and balance

Walking sometimes requires the placement of feet in positions that compromise feelings of stability. It happens almost every day if you walk in cities, on trails, or even down the street. There are dogs on leashes that get entangled, uneven streets, and curbs that sometimes appear out of nowhere (especially if your head is down looking at your phone). Navigating the environment and maintaining the ability to balance in a dynamic way is a part of everyday life.

When certain activities become challenging or, worse, cause fear, it's natural to begin avoiding situations that require those activities. In this case, people experiencing fear around dynamic balance may begin avoiding uneven streets, narrow stairways, or trails. I mentioned earlier research on the elderly has shown anxiety and balance are often correlated; put more simply, as confidence in balance and stability decreases, anxiety increases (Salzman 2010; Gufoni et al. 2005). This can create a snowball effect, leading to social isolation and low self-confidence. This affects emotional well-being and takes away the ability to enjoy – and experience – the benefits of the natural setting. Nature has a number of psychological benefits, including feeling less depressed, less stressed, and more alive (Morita et al. 2007). It should be no surprise that as the ability to feel confident navigating the world decreases, anxiety and depression increase.

The next three exercises can be performed near a wall until confidence improves. Remember, one of the keys to creating successful movement experiences is establishing high levels of neuroception in the individual. This is particularly important if the student is new to balance work and feels a sense of insecurity around how their feet interact with the ground.

Exercise
Stepping over obstacles

Set up four to six obstacles in a line. They can be of varying heights and sizes. Stand facing the obstacles, so the obstacles are in a line directly in front of you (Figure 6.6).

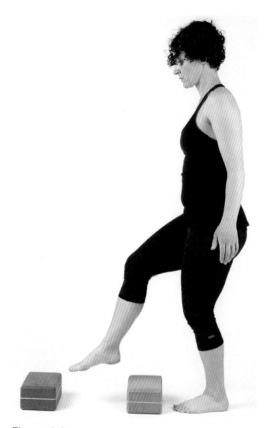

Figure 6.6

Walk over the obstacles going forward. Walk over the obstacles going backward. Walk over the obstacles going sideways.

Things to consider and observe

- Where do the eyes look? Do they look down at the feet or do they look straight ahead?

- What strategy is used to lift the leg? Does the pelvis hike to lift the leg? Does the hip lift the leg? Does the lift come from the foot?

- Is the student breathing?

- Does the person begin walking with the same leg? If so, which leg leaves the ground first?

- Does the student go quickly over the obstacles or slowly? What happens if the student changes their speed? Is it more or less smooth?

The strategy a person uses to lift their leg can be the difference between a leg that feels like feathers and a leg that feels like lead. Think of it this way: when you lift your elbow up so it's even with your shoulder, is it easier to do it by shrugging the shoulder up as you lift the elbow, or when your shoulder stays down? When it stays down, right? When the leg lifts, creating efficiency is similar. If the student's strategy is to hike the hip to lift the leg, that's kind of like hiking the shoulder to lift the elbow – it's more work and makes the limb feel heavier.

An easy way to teach hip flexion is to place the left fingers in the left hip crease. Bend the left knee. You will feel the crease below your fingers begin to deepen. This is hip flexion.

Now, try this. Keep the fingers in the same place, but move the left hand side of the pelvis up toward the left ribs. The left hip might lift, but there won't be much change in the crease beneath the fingertips. This is lateral flexion of the pelvis, the same movement that happens when a student's hip hikes to initiate the movement of lifting the leg.

Hiking the pelvis is a necessary action of human walking, so the goal isn't for the student to eliminate it from their movement repertoire altogether, but for some people it couples with hip flexion, which means the only way the person can flex the hip is by hiking the pelvis. It's difficult to feel; many people don't realize hip hiking is their strategy for initiating leg movement until they have spent some time understanding what hip hiking is. The pelvis oscillates during walking, with the two sides performing opposite actions in unison. This means one side of the pelvis is laterally flexing while the other side is moving down. These motions are performed as the pelvis is rotating, which if you remember from earlier means walking is a tri-planar movement.

If the student struggles with lifting the leg without hiking the pelvis first, in addition to making the leg heavy, what are some other issues this habitual strategy may cause? It can lead to discomfort in the lower side of

Case study

A woman was referred to me for a basic strength and conditioning program to help with pain she was having in her hip. The discomfort was actually in her gluteal region (the area on the outside of the pelvis) and had become so much of a nuisance that she was limiting how much time she spent walking. Stairs, in particular, were challenging and uncomfortable.

I noticed during our first session that when she lifted the leg, the pelvis on that side swung out to the side. During our second session, I had her walk over shallow bolsters, an exercise I commonly use to teach people to lift their feet. "I am getting pain in my hip when I do this," she said.

I had her come into a standing position and place her fingers in her hip crease, as described above. Once she understood the motion, I had her walk over the bolsters again, using the action she had just learned.

As she finished, tears began to stream down her cheeks. "What's wrong?" I asked.

"It doesn't hurt."

Pain is frustrating and exhausting, and often has no obvious cause. Sometimes, a little bit of awareness can make all of the difference.

the back. We will cover this more extensively in Chapters 8 and 9 on the spine and the pelvis, but, for right now, just know that if the student has discomfort with obstacle courses and their strategy for hip flexion is actually hip hiking, until you teach the student how to differentiate between the two movements, actively lifting the leg may exacerbate sensations of discomfort. Learning to differentiate the actions of lateral flexion of the pelvis and hip flexion will result in more mobility and freedom, both in the hips and in the pelvis.

Exercise
Stepping between two objects

Place two objects approximately a leg's distance apart. Stand to the left of the back object, so the front object is in front of you on your left.

Reach your right foot forward, until it is in line with the front object. Slowly, set the right foot down and transfer weight to the right foot, lifting the left leg. Pause for a moment, and then slowly set the left foot down. Transfer weight back and forth, from the left leg to the right leg three or four times and then switch legs (Figures 6.7 and 6.8).

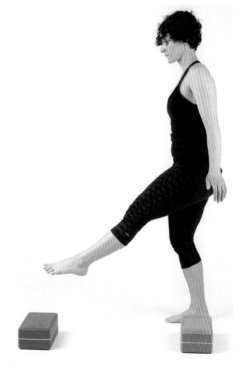

Figure 6.7

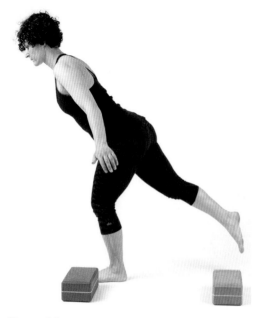

Figure 6.8

Things to consider and observe

- Was the reaching leg able to find the ground with control? Or did it look choppy?

- Did the jaw clench or did the jaw stay loose?

- What happened with the breath?

- What happened when the weight was transferred to the back foot? Did the back foot angle or did it point relatively forward?

- Was one side easier than the other?

- What did the arms do?

Transferring weight is a basic aspect of gait. During reaching exercises, to maximize efficiency while the center of mass is changing locations, integrating the arms into the movement will help to maintain stability. Students who are more rigid will initially struggle with figuring out ways their arms can help them. Instead of telling students

how to reach their arms, ask them, "What happens if you let your arms be part of the movement?" This gives them an opportunity to focus their attention, use intrinsic feedback, and self-organize. Some people may find it easier to reach their arms forward, some out to the side, some backward. None of these are wrong, and once the student becomes comfortable integrating the arms into the movement, you can suggest the arms reach in a different way, so the student can see how different variations feel.

If the student externally rotates the back foot when transferring weight back, this tells you something about their stabilization strategy. The external rotation of the back foot will affect the position of the pelvis by externally rotating and extending the same side hemipelvis. This isn't bad; it's certainly a way to accomplish the task, and if the student is aware the foot externally rotates, that indicates the student has the ability to perform the skill differently if they choose. On the other hand, if the student is unable to feel the external rotation of the back foot, that indicates the movement is habitual. Giving the student more options or suggestions for how the back foot can be placed on the floor may improve efficiency.

When you ask students to perform "normal" daily activities, like taking a large step, in ways that are awkward or unusual, the next time a large step is taken in a normal way it will feel easier. Learning occurs from performing the familiar in an unfamiliar way. The brain is very good at processing what works well and avoiding what doesn't for regular daily activities.

When people are never exposed to doing familiar movements in novel ways, there is nothing to learn from. It's kind of like assuming the chocolate cake recipe you have been making for the last 20 years is the best chocolate cake recipe that exists. If you were to try some other recipes, you would get new ideas and the recipe would evolve. Sure, there may be times when the new recipe isn't as good as the original recipe, but there might be something about the recipe you like so you keep that one small thing to use next time and disregard the rest. Movement is the same – in order to keep evolving and learning, it requires a willingness to make the familiar unfamiliar.

Exercise

Single-leg reaching

Set a timer for 60 seconds. If you are comfortable standing on one leg in the middle of the room, stand on your right leg. If that doesn't sound like a good idea, place yourself near a wall that you can use for balance.

Reach the left foot in front of you. Reach it behind you. Reach it to the right. Reach it to the left. Reach the left foot to as many different places as you can think of, setting the foot down as needed. Imagine you are reaching toward an object you really want to touch. See if you can reach the foot without looking down at it and let the right leg (your standing leg) be responsive, not rigid. How does that feel (Figures 6.9 and 6.10)?

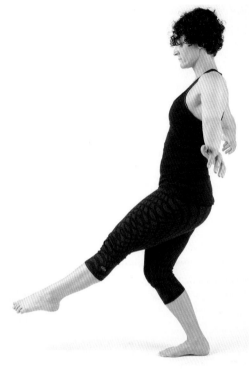

Figure 6.10

When the timer goes off, reset the timer and switch legs.

Things to consider and observe

- Was one side easier than the other?

- How did it feel to reach in different directions? Was one direction easier than the others? Was one direction more challenging?

- Did the torso respond to the movement? What about the standing leg?

This type of exercise focuses attention, teaching dynamic balance in a way that doesn't require input from the teacher. Giving people space to learn, especially with more challenging tasks, improves the likelihood of skill transference and skill retention. These types of drills

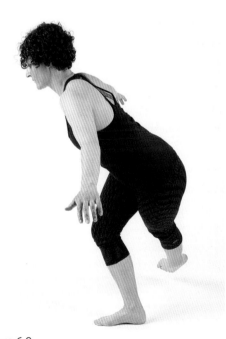

Figure 6.9

are also usually fun for the student – increasing confidence in balance and stability also increases a sense of resilience.

All of the exercises described above require information from the visual and vestibular system. If you notice a student has a specific tendency with the head, such as looking down or cocking the head to one side while performing challenging movements, improving neck mobility and introducing drills that require hand–eye coordination, such as ball throwing or aiming for reaching the hands toward specific objects in various positions, can help the student integrate the visual system more effectively during balance work.

After a lecture recently, I was taking an Uber back to the airport. We chatted about him for a while as I peppered him with questions regarding his driving career. Eventually, he turned the questioning to me, curious why I was there. I told him it was for work. A few more questions ensued, until he asked if I would mind sharing the topic of my lecture. "Exercise recommendations for mental health symptoms," I responded, hoping I wasn't boring him (always a concern, when you teach movement and fitness for a living).

His interest was obviously piqued, and I could see him working to formulate his next question. "What is one thing that most people would find surprising about the information you shared?"

"Poor balance and anxiety are often correlated."

"My mom is really fearful. Maybe I should pay attention to how she walks and see if she's unsteady at all?"

Based on our conversation, I guesstimated he was in his late fifties or early sixties, which meant his mom was probably in her eighties. "You should absolutely pay attention to how steady your mom is. You may be surprised what you see."

Balance is an integration of the neuromuscular system and affects neuroception and the ability to navigate the environment confidently and securely. Implementing

short bouts of dynamic balance training can make a profound impact on emotional and physical well-being, creating stability, confidence, and maybe even inciting playfulness as students begin to explore tasks in a dynamic, unspecified way. Even tasks that seem simple, like getting up and down off the floor in a variety of ways, require an integration of the visual, vestibular, and proprioception systems. Improving embodiment requires enhancing the integration of all of the systems of the physical body, not just control of the musculoskeletal system.

References

Al-Aama T (2014) Falls in the elderly. Canadian Family Physician 60 (3) 225.

Bart O, Bar-Haim Y, Weizman E, Levin M, Sadeh A, and Mintz M (2009) Balance treatment ameliorates anxiety and increases self-esteem in children with comorbid anxiety and balance disorder. Research in Developmental Disabilities 30 (3) 486–495.

Bondolfi G, Jermann F, Van der Linden M, Gex-Fabry M, Bizzini L, Rougent BW, Myers-Arrazola L, Gonzalez C, Segal Z, Aubry J-M, and Bertschy G (2010) Depression relapse prophylaxis with Mindfulness-Based Cognitive Therapy: Replication and extension in the Swiss health care system. Journal of Affective Disorders 122 (3) 224–231.

Carmeli E (2015) Anxiety in the elderly can be a vestibular problem. Frontiers in Public Health 3 216.

Davids K, Button C, Araujo D, Renshaw I, and Hristovski R (2006) Movement models from sports provide representative task constraints for studying adaptive behavior in human movement systems. Adaptive Behavior 14 (1) 73–95.

Dichgans J, Bizzi E, Morasso P, and Tagliasco V (1973) Mechanisms underlying recovery of eye–head coordination following bilateral labyrinthectomy in monkey. Experimental Brain Research 18 (5) 548–562.

Diehl D and Pidcoe P (2006) Gaze stabilization strategies during voluntary head movements: The relationship to fall recovery. Journal of Neurologic Physical Therapy 30 (4) 200.

Fujino M, Ueda Y, Mizuhara H, Saiki J, and Nomura M (2018) Open monitoring meditation reduces the involvement of brain regions related to memory function. Nature 8 (9,968) 1–10.

Goldin PR and Gross JJ (2010) Effects of mindfulness-based stress reduction (MBSR) on emotion regulation in social anxiety disorder. Emotion 10 (1) 83–91.

Grecucci A, De Pisapia N, Kusalagnaana T, Paladino MP, Venuti P, and Job R (2015) Baseline and strategic effects behind mindful emotion regulation: Behavioral and physiological investigation. PLoS ONE 10 (1) e0116541.

Gufoni M, Guidetti G, Nuti D, Pagnini P, Vicini C, Tinelli C, and Mira E (2005) The relationship between cognitive impairment, anxiety-depression symptoms and balance and spatial orientation complaints in the elderly. Acta otorhinolaryngologica Italica: organo ufficiale della Societa italiana di otorinolaringologia e chirurgia cervico-facciale [Official Journal of the Italian Society of Otorhinolaryngology – Head and Neck Surgery] 3 (25) 12–21.

Han HI, Song HS, and Kim JS (2011) Vestibular rehabilitation therapy: Review of indications, mechanisms, and key exercises. Journal of Clinical Neurology 7 (4) 184–196.

Kim D-W and Kim T-H (2018) Effects of abdominal hollowing and abdominal bracing during side-lying hip abduction on the lateral rotation and muscle activity of the pelvis. Journal of Exercise Rehabilitation 14 (2) 226–230.

Li ZM (2006) Functional degrees of freedom. Motor Control 10 (4) 301–310.

Magill RA (1994) The influence of augmented feedback on skill learning depends on characteristics of the skill and the learner. Quest 46 314–327.

McCorry LM (2007) Physiology of the autonomic nervous system. American Journal of Pharmaceutical Education 71 (4) 78.

Mehta R, Cannella M, Henry SM, Smith S, Giszster S, and Silfies SP (2017) Trunk postural muscle timing is not compromised in low back pain patients clinically diagnosed with movement coordination impairments. Motor Control 21 (2) 133–157.

Menz HB (2015) Biomechanics of the aging foot and ankle: A mini-review. Gerontology 61 381–388.

Morita E, Fukuda S, Nagano J, Hamajima N, Yamamoto H, Iwai Y, Nakashima T, Ohira H, and Shirakawa T (2007) Psychological effects of forest environments on healthy adults: Shinrin-yoku (forest-air bathing, walking) as a possible method of stress reduction. Public Health 121 (1) 54–63.

Peeters LHC, Kingma I, Faber GS, van Died JH, and de Grott JM (2018) Trunk, head and pelvis interactions in healthy children when performing seated daily arm tasks. Experimental Brain Research 236 (7) 2,023–2,036.

Proske U and Gandevia SC (2012) The proprioceptive senses: Their roles in signaling body shape, body position and movement, and muscle force. Physiological Reviews 92 (4) 1,651–1,697.

Purves D, Augustine GJ, Fitzpatrick D, Katz LC, LaMantia A-S, McNamara JO, and Williams SM (eds) (2001) Chapter 14, Vestibular system, in Neuroscience, 2nd edn. Sunderland, MA: Sinauer Associates. Available: https://www.ncbi.nlm.nih.gov/books/NBK10819/.

Rahimi A and Abadi ZE (2012) The effects of anxiety on balance parameters in young female university students. Iranian Journal of Psychiatry 7 (4) 176–179.

Salzman B (2010) Gait and balance disorders in older adults. American Family Physician 82 (1) 61–68.

Shefer S, Gordon C, Avraham KB, and Mintz M (2015) Balance deficit enhances anxiety and balance training decreases anxiety in vestibular mutant mice. Behavioral Brain Research 276 76–83.

Stoelben KJV, Pappas E, and Mota CB (2019) Lower extremity joint moments throughout gait at two speeds more than 4 years after ACL reconstruction. Gait Posture 70 347–354.

Stonerock GL, Hoffman BM, Smith PJ, and Blumenthal JA (2015) Exercise as treatment for anxiety: Systematic review and analysis. Annals of Behavioral Medicine 49 (4) 542–556.

Sunaryadi Y (2017) Relative frequency of augmented feedback and motor skill learning. IOP conference series: Materials science and engineering 180. Available: https://doi.org/10.1088/1757-899X/180/1/012229.

Wulf G (2007) Attention and motor skill learning. Champaign, IL: Human Kinetics.

Case study

An 82-year-old client came in to see me after traveling for a few months. He was having significant back pain with nerve pain radiating down the leg. It started after an enthusiastic bout of shoveling snow, an activity he hadn't done in several years. His trainer back home had him do child's pose and bridging, his physical therapist suggested pressing his torso up into extension, and he was frustrated because everything seemed to be making the pain worse, not better.

I gave him some gentle breathing exercises and had him use a ball between his knees to create a little bit of movement in his hips by gently pressing his knees into it and relaxing, which he verified didn't cause an increase in symptoms. When he left, he didn't feel worse, and he felt a teeny bit better. I suggested using the ball exercise in the morning to see if it helped his discomfort upon waking.

The ball squeezes in the morning gave him relief when he first woke up, but he wasn't making progress as quickly as he wanted. I suggested seeing a doctor, and he decided to make an appointment at Stanford with a back surgeon.

A magnetic resonance imaging (MRI) scan showed a disc herniation at L4–L5, consistent with his symptoms. He decided to schedule surgery.

I continued working with him twice a week, carefully monitoring what caused nerve pain and staying away from movements and exercises that caused an increase in discomfort. Over time, I gradually increased reps, paying careful attention to position, and I always had him finish with breathing so that he walked out feeling relaxed. His symptoms were improving, and he was able to do more and more without pain. But the nerve discomfort would still flare up occasionally, and it was at its worst first thing in the morning. I told him discs heal and he was improving, but he was determined to move forward with the surgery.

Exactly three months after the onset of injury, the day before he was supposed to go in for surgery, he woke up and the pain was gone. He canceled surgery, and he's been pain free ever since.

When an area is first injured, it's wise to avoid the activities that cause sharp pain. This is true of any body part; the back is no different. Forcing positions or movements that cause pain doesn't help the healing process; in fact, it may slow things down.

However, if it's been longer than three months, physical therapy has been successfully completed, and there is something a student really wants to be able to do, the techniques and concepts discussed throughout this chapter will help the student move in the right direction. Slowly exposing the student to different positions in different ways, monitoring how they respond, and gradually building strength and flexibility will enable the student to eventually be able to do the things they want to do, when they want to do them.

There is a strong chance you will encounter a student with low back or neck pain at some point during your career. Research suggests 80% of people in the US will experience low back pain at some point in their lives (Freburger et al. 2009). Fortunately, low back pain usually clears up within a few months, regardless of the intervention used. This means if chiropractic/acupuncture/massage/going on vacation is the preferred therapeutic modality of the student and the student thinks it works, the student should absolutely do the helpful thing; it is also worthwhile to note the likelihood that the student would have improved without the intervention is high. It is entirely plausible that my client in the case study above would have felt better had he not seen me; seeing me made him feel better about his situation and improved his sense of resilience, both of which improved his mood and emotional well-being while he was healing.

continued

A common reason people visit doctors is for nonspecific low back pain (NSLBP). NSLBP is back pain that is coming from an unspecified cause, other than spinal degeneration. One potential cause of NSLBP is a sedentary lifestyle – lack of physical activity reduces the ability of the vertebral disc to maintain its normal water concentration. This influences the development of degeneration (Citko et al. 2018). Movement provides nourishment to the tissues; in fact, one of the worst things you can do for your back if it hurts is lie in bed and not move. After the first 72 hours following acute injury, movement is an effective way to improve blood flow to the tissues, which is necessary for healing (Chinn & Hertel 2010). (For the first 72 hours, #netflixandchill is perfectly okay. Acute injuries and trauma make movement uncomfortable, and relaxing while tissues are inflamed initially isn't a bad thing.)

As a movement practitioner, it's important during the early stages of tissue healing to implement gentle movement as tolerated. A trick I have used over the years is to work on areas far away from the injury site. This not only reminds the student there are other body parts that still work, it also reduces the perception of threat for the student. When the student realizes there are movements they can perform that don't cause pain, they usually become more willing to try movements that require integration of body parts closer to the site of injury. It's critical to maintain open communication – I usually tell the student in a relaxed way, "If this causes any discomfort, just let me know. It means I have to re-route."

Disc herniations, which are defined as a protrusion of the middle part of the disc through the hard outer casing, are also called slipped or ruptured discs. Though the terminology used to describe this condition sounds scary, in a large research review of low back imaging in asymptomatic people, 84% of people aged 80 or older had a disc protrusion. To be clear, these individuals had no low back pain (Brinjiki et al. 2014). This suggests disc herniations shouldn't be feared, and while they can contribute to the onset of pain, they aren't a guarantee that pain will be present (Steffens et al. 2014).

Another important thing to remember about disc herniations is that tissues heal, including disc protrusions. When imaging was performed on subjects months after the initial disc injury, it showed a decrease in the size of herniation, and, in some cases, the disc protrusion completely disappeared. Researchers suggest in many cases conservative treatment, including movement, should be used to treat symptomatic disc herniations (Bozzao et al. 1992; Ellenberg et al. 1993).

I have worked with a handful of people directly after disc herniations obtained while sneezing, shoveling snow, and colonoscopies. Directly after the injury, all of them exhibited poor motor control and poor proprioception, just like you would expect with any injury. In all of the cases, I played what felt like a detective, figuring out which moves were sensitive and where their perceived center of balance was. When an injury affects the center of the body, it shouldn't come as a surprise that the student's ability to discern the center of mass is often altered, impacting proprioception and the ability to feel balanced (Parkhurst & Burnett 1994).

The key to healing is to initially avoid the positions that cause pain, go slowly, and introduce loaded movements gradually. Instead of three sets of eight loaded squats, for instance, I may program one set of loaded squats, see how the person responds, slowly adding in sets and reps during subsequent sessions. Sometimes load feels better than no load; sometimes bodyweight feels better. Paying attention to position and using drills that improve proprioception of the torso and spine is important; so is eventually introducing mobility to the areas above and below the herniation. If the herniation was at the level of L4–L5, teaching upper thoracic and isolated hip mobility as tolerated four weeks

continued

after the injury is good for tissue health. Remember, after an acute injury, the student should be under the care of a physician and physical therapist. The job of the movement professional is to act as an adjunct to therapy, improving strength and mobility throughout the entire system and helping the student regain confidence in their physical abilities. As long as the practitioner creates a restorative movement to work ratio that is high at first, giving the student an opportunity to respond and acclimate to load as tolerated, the practitioner can work with the client in a gentle, safe way.

Injuries or irritation in the spinal region are scary for people. Many equate it with the potential for serious damage and pain. The good news is the spine and the ligaments and muscles that support it are designed to withstand force, keeping you upright and moving in a variety of ways, every day. In fact, every time you take a step while walking, there is a ground reaction force that's anywhere from 50% of your bodyweight to your full bodyweight. When you run, the ground reaction force can be up to three times your

bodyweight (Matijevich et al. 2018). The body evolved to deal with these forces in an effective and efficient way, and the back is no exception.

It is important to note low back pain can be a symptom of more serious issues, such as benign cysts that are irritating a nerve or malignant tumors (Mabry et al. 2014; Fattahi et al. 2014). If pain persists with little to no improvement, encourage the student to seek medical advice.

In Chapter 1, I talked about mindset and how people think about their bodies. If you are working with someone who has dealt with low back pain, it is important that you don't describe their core as weak or suggest their low back pain is a result of lazy glute muscles or a faulty breathing pattern. Language around the body and the fact that it is strong, capable, and can withstand large amounts of load is critical for reducing fear and anxiety around movement. Perhaps most importantly, language can be used to remind the student the body is part of them. It's not a separate entity and how they view their bodies reflects how they view themselves and is an important aspect of the healing process.

Sensitization and habituation

I mentioned sensitization earlier, but to quickly re-cap, if there is a position that consistently causes the sensation of pain even after the acute injury should technically be healed, the student is sensitized to the position. Researchers suggest sensitization happens at the level of the central nervous system (CNS). Nociceptor sensory fibers are louder than the situation requires, and the amount of neurons in the CNS pain pathway is increased. The combination of loud nociceptors and the perception that a specific movement is associated with pain means that when the student approaches the painful position, pain happens (Woolf 2011).

It is not uncommon for individuals with persistent low back pain to demonstrate less movement variability and

complexity (Gizzi et al. 2019). What this means is instead of having 20 strategies for picking up a bag of groceries, the person has one strategy for picking up the bag of groceries. The person picks up the groceries exactly the same way, every time.

Over the years, I have worked with a number of people who have become sensitized to their movement habits. This results in pain every time they do a specific activity, like sitting in their car, standing, or picking an object up off the ground. When the movement is approached a different way, the pain disappears. This may require creativity on the practitioner's part since not every intervention or approach to a different movement will work for every person.

One thing that happens with any focused movement practice, whether it's a mind–body practice like yoga, a gymnastics-based bodyweight program, or a strength training program, is options for movement increase in sedentary individuals, so simply gaining strength and moving more will increase strength and decrease symptoms. If the student is already very physically active and is struggling with a chronic pain issue, usually if you look closely enough, you will see a lack of variability in some aspect of the individual's movement. In physical therapy, the solution is usually to strengthen the muscles that oppose the person's movement habit. (This is the philosophy behind a lot of postural correction systems. If the person habitually moves one way, strengthening the opposite position will give the student an option of moving differently.) Since we learned earlier that posture isn't necessarily indicative of pain, this solution may be outdated and may not work for everyone. A better solution may be to gradually increase exposure to different positions using a variety of tools, including improved proprioception, strength, and mobility.

Let's look at sitting more specifically, since there are lots of ideas regarding how a person "should" sit. Many people have a preconceived idea that slouching is bad for the back, so they purposefully try to sit up straight. After a few minutes, they experience discomfort so they slouch, and when they catch themselves slouching they go into a state of panic, because they read slouching is sure to cause imminent damage, making their pain worse, so they go back to sitting up straight. The cycle continues until their low back is screaming. Since they were sitting the "right" way but still had discomfort, they conclude sitting is bad for their back.

Our bodies are designed for variable movement, so subtle shifting to change positions while sitting is a good thing. The good news is that it's okay to slouch while sitting if it reduces discomfort in the back. It's still important to shift occasionally, but there is no reason to force students to sit up "straight" if it hurts.

Straight is, of course, relative. Many people perceive sitting up straight as thrusting their ribs forward and shoving their shoulders down and back. Often, simply relaxing the ribs down and letting the shoulders relax

forward create instant changes in a person's experience. I was working with a client recently, teaching her how to perform a seated, one-arm row without thrusting her ribs forward when she said, "I have been to a lot of trainers and fitness professionals. How come you are the first person to help me with this?" If you always prescribe the same cues, regardless of which movement modality you study, it's important to ask yourself why you use the cues you use and what happens if you cue the movement differently. How does that change the student's experience?

Sometimes, the opposite is true and people are sensitive to slouching. In this case, asking the person to change the position of the pelvis, so they are sitting more on top of the sitting bones rather than behind them, results in less discomfort.

One of the great things about you and the people you work with is that you are living, breathing organisms with the capacity to learn. The entire system can learn, which means people can (eventually) learn to be in the position that's currently uncomfortable if the position is approached with curiosity and patience.

There is a concept called graded exposure therapy. If you have ever been in therapy for an anxiety disorder or you or a loved one has a peanut allergy, you may be familiar with it. Essentially, the subject is gradually exposed to the thing that causes an undesirable reaction, enabling the subject to (hypothetically) build up a tolerance to the threatening movement/behavior/allergen.

Anxiety disorders and food allergies are both associated with triggers. For someone who suffers from social anxiety or claustrophobia, being with a crowd of people in a confined space might well trigger a panic attack, even though the situation is by no means life threatening. Peanuts in some individuals trigger an autoimmune response that can be deadly.

Let's say the thought of public speaking triggers an increase in heart rate, shortness of breath, and causes you to feel like you might pass out or have a heart attack.

The solution isn't to speak in front of 100 people tomorrow; instead, you might try speaking in front of two people you are comfortable with, observing both your initial response and reflecting on how you felt afterwards. Assuming it went okay and, while you felt nervous, there were no negative outcomes as a result of speaking, perhaps next week you would try speaking in front of three people, gradually increasing the number of people and eventually introducing people you don't know into the mix. Over time, you would no longer associate the idea of public speaking (the trigger) with a negative outcome and your anticipatory response to the thought of public speaking would be different (McGuire et al. 2014).

A similar protocol can be used with food allergies, such as peanuts (Lanser et al. 2015). Individuals with severe peanut allergies are given tiny doses of peanuts every day, a mere fraction, so their system is exposed to the potentially "harmful" substance in such a small dose that it doesn't cause a severe allergic reaction. Gradually, over a very long period of time, the amount of peanut given increases. This is all done under medical supervision, just like the scenario above is done under the guidance of a psychologist. These aren't the types of treatments to try on yourself without the help of a trained professional. Eventually, the individual can be exposed to the trace amounts of peanuts often found in restaurants or packaged food because their sensitivity to the trigger has lessened.

The body works the same way. If someone experiences pain performing a specific movement for no physiological reason, opportunities to repetitively approach the sensitive situation and then move away from it can be introduced, assuming the basic principles of pain science have been explained. If an individual expects an action to hurt and that it will cause tissue damage, the action will likely hurt. Understanding that no tissue damage will occur by approaching the position in a variety of ways is important for the student's emotional well-being. The trigger is the sensitive position. The intervention is to approach the position, stopping right before discomfort sets in. Over time, the place where the discomfort sets in will shift, until, eventually, it disappears (Nijs et al. 2014).

It's well documented that there are structural changes in symptomatic lower extremity tendinopathies; loading the area causes structural adaptations and improvements in function, reducing pain. Increasing load too soon places soft tissues at risk for injury. (An easy way to remember this is that load shouldn't exceed capacity. Capacity, in this case, is the ability of the tissues to withstand the stress placed upon them.) The goal of the practitioner becomes to increase tolerance by loading the tissues gradually, giving the neuromuscular system and the skeletal system an opportunity to adapt before adding more load. This also improves the student's confidence by reminding them the area that is experiencing discomfort is actually strong and can withstand stress (Zellmer et al. 2019).

Practical application

Before exploring specific exercises, let's integrate the concepts of variability and habituation into a practical exploration.

Find a chair you can sit in so your feet rest comfortably on the ground (not a problem for most of the people reading this, I know, but as someone who is 5'1" with very short legs, I can attest that not all furniture is designed so the feet actually touch the ground for those of us who are not well endowed in the height department).

Set a timer for 3 minutes. Stand up. Sit back down. Take a moment to think about how you just stood up from the chair.

Spend the rest of the allotted time standing up and sitting down different ways. Try to make each attempt at standing up different in some way than the preceding one.

When the timer goes off, take a moment to reflect. Were there any variations you stumbled across that you found interesting? Were there any that were challenging? Did you learn anything about yourself?

Standing up and sitting down is an excellent example of something most of us do often during the day, without thinking about how we perform the movement. It's habitual, which is good – it enables us to change positions quickly, without too much effort. I often teach a variation of this exercise when I lecture, and it's always interesting to watch people pause for a brief second while they figure out how they might stand up differently than they just did. As a movement teacher, teaching people to stand up and sit down in many different ways is not only a fun exercise; it also gives people options for a daily, habitual task.

Exercise

Pelvis awareness in seated: rocking from side to side

Come into a seated position in a chair with your feet flat on the floor and your hands resting by your side. Find the place where the sitting bones, the two bones on the bottom of the pelvis, are resting on the chair. Gently rock to the right, so the right side of the pelvis is weighted more heavily than the left. Gently rock to the left, so the left side of the pelvis is weighted more heavily than the right. Go back and forth between these two positions six to eight times and return to center.

Variation

You can also try rolling around the sitting bones, as though you were making a circle that goes forward, right, back, and to the left of the sitting bones. If you try this, make sure you change directions and see how it feels going the other way as well.

Things to consider and observe

- Did the knees move or the feet lift while you were moving the pelvis?

- Which direction was easier for you, going to the right or to the left?

- Are you able to feel both sitting bones, or does one feel heavier than the other?

- Did the torso and head move as well, or is movement isolated at the pelvis?

You will notice that some of the observations, like keeping the knees still, were not part of the original instructions. That's because it's interesting to observe a person's interpretation and movement strategies without giving them too many things to consider. The next time the student attempts the same movement, you can ask the student to keep the knees or head still as a way to direct the student's attention. When clients ask me if they were doing it "wrong" before, I respond, "No. I am just giving you an alternative way to try it." Good teaching is done in layers: create awareness, offer one option at a time, and invite the student to become curious about movement.

The above exercise is an example of a gentle movement that can be used to gradually expose the body to different pelvis positions. If the same movement were repeated again, chances are high it would be easier and the movement would be more coordinated. The nervous system takes stock of positions that may be potentially painful by limiting range of motion. Once the new position is deemed safe, the nervous system relaxes, enabling more freedom of movement.

A clearer example of this is the stretch reflex. When someone is initially placed in a position or stretch that feels tight, the experience of the sensation is fairly intense. Depending on the area being stretched and the individual's basic overall flexibility, that experience can range anywhere from "that feels like a nice stretch," to "I think the muscle is going to rip off of the bone."

There are specialized mechanoreceptors in muscle fibers that detect stretch (Purves et al. 2001). When a student moves into a position they haven't been in since they were seven, these specialized mechanoreceptors send really loud warning signs in the form of sensation, letting them know this position is foreign and potentially harmful.

If the student were to do something else, approaching the same position again 3 minutes later, there would be less sensation and, more than likely, the student would be able to move into the position more comfortably and with a fuller range of motion. It's not that the student suddenly became more flexible (unfortunately – if only it were that easy). The nervous system simply adjusted sensation based on feedback from the previous experience.

Case study

A long-time client of mine suffered a severe disc herniation in her neck while she was sleeping. She woke up with nerve pain all of the way down the left arm, nausea, and a general feeling of being unwell.

She had surgery a few days later, which included removing what looked like crab meat where the disc had herniated and a cervical disc fusion. Six weeks after surgery, she resumed exercise with me.

I worked on gentle movements with her to restore motion in her arm that had been affected by the nerve pain. The pain was gone, but the arm still felt foreign to her. In order to improve movement through her mid back, I had her hold her arms in front of her with her palms facing each other and the elbows bent, moving the right elbow under the left and then the left elbow under the right, with the eventual goal of the top elbow resting above the bottom elbow, in the crook of the arm.

The first time she did it, the left elbow barely moved. The elbows remained far apart, and the action was extremely challenging. After four weeks, she was approaching the midline. They still didn't touch, but they were much closer and the sensation she felt the very first time she had tried it was significantly reduced.

It's now been years since her surgery and she can perform the movement without any trouble or discomfort. A huge part of restoring function after a physical trauma like surgery is trying different movements. If they don't work the first time, wait a few days or a week and ask the student to try it again. Repeated exposure in a thoughtful way and in a safe setting is what creates the opportunity for the muscles and the brain to respond through adaptation and learning.

The anatomy of the spine

The head sits on top of the first cervical vertebra in the spinal column, which is known as the atlas. This vertebra differs from the others because it lacks a vertebral body and spinous process, and, as a result, is ring shaped. The neck region of the spine comprises seven vertebrae, which naturally curve forward. Interestingly, all mammals have the same number – from the giraffe to my small Maltese dog. (Obviously, the sizes of the vertebrae differ greatly depending on the species.) The cervical, thoracic and, lumbar spine usually consists of 24 vertebrae. This number can vary, however, because anatomical variations exist. In fact it has been suggested that between 10% and 17% of adults have some kind of spinal abnormality. Most commonly this manifests as an extra vertebra in the lumbar region, but it is also possible to either gain or lose one of the thoracic vertebra in association with an extra or missing pair of ribs (Yan et al. 2018).

The second cervical vertebra also has a special name. It's called the axis and it allows you to rotate the head right and left. The axis has a special bony projection called the dens that attaches to the atlas and allows the second vertebrae to serve as an axis of rotation, hence the name (Menon 2019).

Running lengthwise between the cervical vertebrae and exiting out the cervical vertebrae are nerves. These nerves travel throughout the head, neck, shoulders, arms, and fingers and are an information superhighway, providing all of the information I have been discussing with regards to sensation to the brain and telling the muscles what needs to happen to move the joints. Another way to say this is the nerves in the cervical spine innervate the head, neck, arms, and shoulders.

The cervical spine nerves also innervate the diaphragm, which, if you remember from Chapter 3, is the muscle that contracts and relaxes every time you breathe (Davies 2010). Interesting, isn't it, that the nerves that provide sensory information and motor control to the shoulders and neck also provide sensory and motor information to the muscle of breathing? A mnemonic that is frequently used to remember which area innervates the diaphragm is "C3, 4, 5 keeps the diaphragm alive."

A number of muscles attach the head to the cervical vertebrae, allowing the head to move in a variety of ways. The head can move up and down, rotate from side to side, and laterally flex. It can also reach up toward the ceiling, reach away from the ceiling, and glide anteriorly and posteriorly. Every time the head moves, the vertebrae in the cervical spine respond to disperse the force generated by the skull, which weighs 10 to 12 pounds. When you walk straight ahead, the gaze stays relatively forward unless balance is compromised or vision is impaired (Cohen 2001; Maslivec et al. 2017). Both of these scenarios alter where the eyes are looking, which changes the position of the head. Remember from Chapter 6 that vision is one of the components of balance; walking requires the base of support to change rapidly, which means maintaining balance is part of staying in an upright, forward position. When proprioception or vision are impaired in some way, how the eyes are used to maintain stability will be affected (Dang et al. 2017).

Below the cervical vertebrae are the thoracic vertebrae, which also happen to be where the ribs attach. The first 10 ribs attach in the front of the torso to the sternum, while the last two ribs are floating, attaching to the 11th and 12th thoracic vertebrae (Safarini & Bordoni 2019). This area is often referred to as the upper and middle back. These vertebrae naturally curve posteriorly, or back, in a subtle way. The nerves in this part of the spine provide control and sensation for the upper back, chest, and abdomen.

The sternum, which happens to be the anterior anchor point for the ribs, is commonly called the breast bone. It has three main parts: the manubrium, the body, and the xiphoid process. The manubrium is the thickest and strongest part of the sternum; the clavicular notch, which is a shallow depression on the upper, lateral part of the manubrium, is where the clavicle meets the sternum at the sternoclavicular joint. The first ribs connect to the manubrium as well (Scheuer & Black 2000).

The manubrium meets the body of the sternum at the sternal angle. This also happens to be where the second rib attaches. The next five ribs (ribs 3–7) attach to the body of the sternum.

The bottom of the sternum is the xiphoid process, a cartilaginous structure earlier in life that becomes ossified during middle age. Multiple muscles attach to the xiphoid process, and it is the anatomical location that coincides with determining where to perform chest compressions during cardiopulmonary resuscitation (CPR) (Anderson & Burns 2018).

Because the first seven ribs attach directly to the sternum, they are classified as true ribs. The costal cartilage of rib 8 attaches to rib 7, the cartilage of rib 9 attaches to rib 8, and the cartilage of rib 10 attaches to rib 9. (If you ever have the opportunity to look at an anatomically correct skeleton, how the ribs attach and the amount of cartilage associated with each rib is worth observing.) The last two ribs are considered false ribs because they don't attach to the sternum at all. Ribs 8–12 are called false ribs due to their lack of direct sternal attachment.

Each thoracic vertebra has costal facets. This is where the ribs attach to the thoracic vertebrae, at the costovertebral joint. Due to the rib attachment on the vertebrae, the thoracic vertebrae have less flexion and extension capabilities than the lumbar vertebrae. It's not that the thoracic vertebrae are unable to flex and extend; they can. It's just not as large a motion as it is in the neighboring parts of the spine.

The middle of the thoracic spine, T5–T8, is capable of large degrees of rotation, while T12 serves as a transitionary vertebra and has similarities in structure to the lumbar vertebrae. This means it's shaped to allow for flexion, extension, and rotation (Waxenbaum & Futterman 2018). Like the cervical vertebrae, lateral flexion also occurs in the thoracic vertebrae.

Below the thoracic vertebrae are the five lumbar vertebrae. These vertebrae curve slightly forward, giving the spine an "s" shaped appearance and making the command "stand up straight" impossible – a well-functioning spine has both mobility, so it can move a variety of ways, and curves, because real spines have curves.

The lumbar vertebral body is larger than the bodies of the cervical and thoracic vertebrae, enabling the lumbar spine to support the weight of the upper body. L5 has the largest vertebral body and creates an angle where it meets the sacrum at the lumbosacral angle. The anatomy of the lumbar vertebrae means it has the largest degree of extension in the spinal column; the vertebrae are well designed for flexion, extension, and lateral flexion, but have less rotation relative to the thoracic vertebrae (Waxenbaum & Futterman 2018).

The nerves in the cervical and thoracic area look like a cord. After the thoracic vertebrae, the spinal cord separates into strands, looking more like a horse's tail, and innervates the buttocks, legs, and feet. Another name for this part of the spinal cord is *cauda equina* and is literally translated as "horse's tail" (Berg & Ashurst 2018).

The fifth lumbar vertebra meets the sacrum, a triangular shaped bone that consists of five vertebrae fused together, at the lumbosacral joint. This joint allows the pelvis to rotate, a movement that takes place every time you walk. The sacrum makes up the back wall of the pelvis, and connects to the pelvis at the sacroiliac joint. It's built to withstand load, and transmits forces from the leg to the torso (Wong & Kiel 2019).

Below the sacrum is one more bone consisting of four fused vertebrae, the coccyx. It moves forward when you sit, acting as a shock absorber. When you rolled your pelvis forward and back in the seated exercise above, you could also have imagined your tail moving between your legs and behind you – it would have elicited the same motion while feeling different.

Practical application: spinal visualization

Set a timer for 3 minutes. Lie down on your back with your legs extended. If that's uncomfortable, bend your knees and place your feet flat on the floor.

Feel the weight of your head against the floor. Visualize where the head connects to the first cervical vertebrae.

Visualize each vertebrae down the spine, the seven cervical vertebrae, 12 thoracic vertebrae, five lumbar vertebrae, sacrum, and coccyx. See if you can feel where the curves change based on the pressure of your spine against the floor.

Go slowly, and if there are areas you can't feel or "see," make a mental note and move on, observing without judging.

When the timer goes off, come into a seated position and feel your spine supporting you. Can you feel more of yourself?

You can also have the student assume the same starting position, but instead of visualizing the vertebrae, ask the student to visualize different spinal movements, asking them to imagine at which place in the spine the movement originates. For instance, if you ask the student to imagine rolling on to their right side, ask the student which parts of the spine participate in the motion. Which part of the spine moves first? Which moves last or doesn't move at all?

Visualization is a form of learning. Based on what you have learned so far, this should make sense. Visualization requires focused attention, self-reflection, and invites curiosity. These are all components of an effective learning intervention. It's also performed in a position that is comfortable and in a safe environment, creating an optimal setting for focusing and learning.

Motor imagery is a term used to describe the mental execution of a movement without any actual movement or muscle activation. Research suggests that imagining a movement activates the same areas of the brain as actually performing the movement (Mulder 2007). If someone has sensation in their low back while rolling onto their side, for instance, tools like motor imagery can be effective for helping the student explore alternative ways to roll through visualization.

Chapter 7

Performing a motor imagery exercise or an awareness exercise in a supine position also allows the brain to integrate the sensory information from the floor regarding the body's position. This may improve both body schema and motor control. Researchers believe the brain's ability to control body movement is related to an individual's body schema (for a more complete overview of this topic, please review Chapter 2) (Morasso et al. 2015).

Exercises involving visualizing specific areas or visualizing movement can be used directly before teaching a related skill or as a way to end a lesson. The reflection required for visualization sometimes works better for students after they have spent time using their body. For some students, movement makes it easier to feel and sense; for others, feeling and sensing makes it easier to move.

Visualizing the spine is another way to color in the body schema. The areas a student struggles to feel or visualize are likely areas that the student struggles to move consciously. Taking the time to practice visualizing and isolating movement at specific parts of the spine improves the likelihood that more of the spine will be integrated into movement, leading to effective dispersal of load throughout the spinal column.

Think of a rubber band. When you stretch a brand new rubber band, it feels like the entire rubber band is stretching. When you stop pulling on the rubber band, it returns to the original position in a uniform way.

If you consistently pull on the same place in the rubber band, that part gets loose. It stops returning to the original position, while other parts of the rubber band remain stiff. The rubber band is no longer dispersing load evenly, which makes the rubber band less springy.

Though this isn't exactly how the spine works, you get the idea – when people consistently move one part of the spine and immobilize the rest, there will be a lot of mobility in one area. The rest of the spine will feel stiff, or stuck.

From an efficiency standpoint, it's beneficial to have movement throughout the spine. It's also beneficial to be able to create what feels like a sense of stillness throughout the spine, though, as noted in Chapter 3, the spine is never completely still. But, the ability to create stiffness is as important as having spinal flexibility and mobility. Spinal stiffness, also thought of as spinal stability, is what allows you to lift heavy objects and create power when you do things like jump or lift the body on to the kitchen counter to put dishes away. The rubber band doesn't yield right away to initiate the movement, but when it does finally move, it returns to the original position. When I am initially assessing clients, I often ask, "Can you create movement in the spine? Where do you feel the movement? And what happens when you try to keep the spine still and move an arm or a leg?"

Spinal stiffness can be taught as a low-threshold strategy or a high-threshold strategy. What do those terms mean?

Let's say you wanted to teach someone how to lift their arm up without moving their spine. You can cue the person to perform the movement in a relaxed manner and ask the person to lift the arm up on the exhale (because of the effects of the exhale on the ribs, this generally works well to dissociate spinal movement from shoulder flexion). You could also have the student lie down on their back and ask the student to initiate the movement from different parts of the arm, taking a more somatic-based approach. "Initiate the lift of the arm from the wrist. Now, initiate the lift from the elbow." Eventually, when you ask the student to lift from the shoulder, usually the movement feels light and easy with minimal torso movement. This can then be translated into standing, and based on what the student just learned about shoulder flexion efficiency, generally there will be little to no movement in the spine. Both lifting on the exhale and initiating the movement from different parts of the arm are examples of a low-threshold strategy, a strategy that is based on the CNS's ability to initiate contraction of the core musculature in a feed-forward manner. This is the strategy you use when you reach for a bag in the car or when you are gesticulating while lecturing. You don't have to interfere with it because it happens automatically; sometimes, movement habits get in the way, creating extra, unnecessary movement. Exercises performed in a relaxed manner with focused awareness can usually re-establish the automaticity of the CNS to create stability.

Exercises that don't require a lot of effort, like lifting the arm, are examples of exercises that can be performed using a low-threshold strategy (Sharma & Kaur 2017).

Another way you could teach the same action is to ask the person to come into a standing position and imagine tension radiating from the belly button, up to the head, down to the toes, and out to the fingers. Keep the sensation of tension radiating throughout your entire body while you lift the right arm up and lower it down. This (obviously) feels different, but accomplishes the exact same thing – the arm lifts up without the spine moving. This is an example of a high-threshold strategy using irradiation. Sherrington's law of irradiation is based on the work of Sir Charles Scott Sherrington (1857–1952), a neurophysiologist who made several contributions to rehabilitative sciences, including defining the term "proprioception" and coining the term "synapse" to describe the actions of reflexes (Pearce 2004).

Irradiation means muscle activation spreads; by generating tension throughout the entire body, all of the muscles that support the torso will be actively participating in the contraction, keeping the spine still while the student lifts the arm (which will feel heavy, because of all of the force being generated throughout the neuromuscular system). Does the student need this much tension to lift their arm? No. Will it make the student stronger? Yes. Is it better than the low-threshold strategy (Gontijo et al. 2012)?

I like to say, "There is no better. Only different" (which my husband likes to quote back to me on occasion, when I am making a bold statement about something being better than something else). The strategy I use depends on the person in front of me. Does the person need more strength? If the answer is yes, a high-threshold strategy is probably what I will teach. If the person is already using a high-threshold strategy of bracing and tensing during most daily activities, then I will teach a low-threshold strategy. Eventually, I want the person who currently isn't very strong to have enough strength that I can teach either strategy, just like I want the tense person to eventually not look like they are using Herculean effort to pick up a pillow. Just like variability is important, so is having the ability to use as much – or as little – force as necessary to complete the task.

When people have basic levels of strength and understand how to move both in a relaxed manner and a more forceful manner, it makes it easier to generate the appropriate amount of force necessary for the task at hand. When I deadlift, I automatically feel my muscles tense as I wrap my hands around the bar. When I lower myself to the floor from a standing position without using my hands, I feel myself relax to respond to the movement. I find individuals who participate in both low-intensity and high-intensity physical activities have a nervous system that's more attuned to dialing force up (or down).

Intervertebral discs

Let's continue looking at the anatomy of the spine. I mentioned that in between each vertebra is a disc, also known as an intervertebral disc. Intervertebral discs are made of cartilage and act as shock absorbers between the vertebrae. The outside of the disc is called the annulus fibrosis, and it's strong; just like a tire is strong enough to support the weight of a car, the annulus fibrosis is strong enough to bear the weight of the vertebrae.

The middle of the disc is made up of the nucleus pulposus (NP). It's more gel-like in consistency and is filled with fluid. It's made primarily of water, and the amount of water in the NP varies throughout the day. When you sleep, the NP is more hydrated; and when you apply load, the disc loses water. As a result, most people are about 10 millimeters shorter by the end of the day. The NP thrives on both activity during the day and rest at night (Cramer 2014).

As noted above, when a disc herniates, the material that makes up the disc becomes disfigured. A portion of the disc (usually the middle) moves beyond the intervertebral space, "bulging" out (Jordan et al. 2009). To recap on earlier, not all disc herniations are symptomatic and, often, with time, discs heal, no longer appearing herniated in imaging (Henmi et al. 2002; Kawaji et al. 2001; Altun & Yuksel 2017).

There are times when herniations are severe and require surgery, but not always. It's important to remember that people are capable of healing and their backs are inherently strong; using the body only makes it stronger.

Exercise

Differentiated cat/cow, directional cueing

Come into a hands-and-knees position or a forearm-and-knees position if you have trouble loading the wrists. Place the elbows under the shoulders and the knees under the hips. Lift the back of the throat to the ceiling and then toward the floor. Go back and forth between the two positions four times, resting as needed.

Now, move the breast bone toward the ceiling and then toward the floor, again, going back and forth between the two positions four times, resting as needed (Figure 7.1).

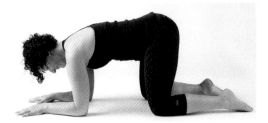

Figure 7.1

Move the lower ribs up toward the ceiling and then toward the floor four times, resting as needed.

Move the belly toward the ceiling and toward the floor four times, resting as needed.

Pretend you have a tail. Move the tail toward the ceiling and toward the floor four times, resting as needed.

Things to consider and observe

- Which sections moved easily?
- Which sections were harder to move?
- Did you feel antsy or frustrated at all? If so, why?
- Were there any places where it felt like muscular work? If so, which areas felt like they were working?
- Did you remember to breathe?

We learned earlier the thoracic spine is less good at flexion and extension than the cervical and lumbar spine. This means isolating movement at the thoracic spine by moving just the breast bone or just the lower ribs is often challenging and possibly frustrating. If the student struggles with isolating the area, it can be helpful to give the student a more externally based task by placing a bolster or foam block on the student's back directly behind the sternum and asking them to move the part of the back touching the object closer to it and away from it. This often makes it more clear which part of the spine should be moving.

If the student can't feel which parts of their spine are moving, video feedback can also be helpful. Film the student performing the task and allow the student to watch the replay before the next attempt. Not everyone likes being filmed, but students who are open to it will reap large benefits.

If there are positions that are particularly challenging, an easy way to begin building more mobility and strength is through isometric contractions. Ask the student to move in and out of the position a few times, exposing the neuromuscular system to the range of motion that feels foreign in a gentle, safe way. Once the student has cycled in and out of the position four to six times, have them hold the weak position for one to two breaths. The isometric contraction builds both strength and proprioception. Focusing on the breath calms the sympathetic nervous system down. In exercises like the one above, if the student focuses on breathing into the area they are isometrically contracting they get the added benefit of more mobility due to the intimate relationship between the diaphragm and the spine.

Exercise
Assessing habits

I don't use a formal assessment tool. I prefer to watch people move and observe their natural tendencies. This, in addition to listening to what they tell me, gives me the information I need to formulate a plan. Below are two assessments I frequently do with new clients to get a sense of their natural way of moving. I cover more assessment ideas in Appendix III.

Lie on your back with your knees bent and your feet flat. Give yourself a hug.

Observe: Which arm is on top (Figure 7.2)?

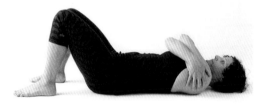

Figure 7.2

Keep the head on the ground and rotate the torso by lifting one shoulder off of the ground. Do this five or six times (Figure 7.3).

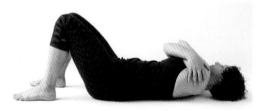

Figure 7.3

Observe: Which direction did you choose to rotate? Did the pelvis move, or the ribs, or both?

Switch the arm that's on top and rotate the other direction five or six times.

Observe: Was this harder or easier?

Stand up. Lift a foot off of the floor, as though you were about to step.

Observe: Which foot did you lift?

People generally rotate initially toward the direction that's more comfortable and generally leave the foot on the ground that's more stable when they are asked to lift a leg. Observing these types of movements can give you an idea of where people perceive their center of mass to be, how people use their feet, and how they use their spines. Creating movement programs that give students opportunities to move their bodies in a way that opposes what they normally do establishes a more resilient system and increases the student's degrees of freedom.

The spine is frequently visualized as a column. However, as noted earlier, the vertebrae that make up the column move independently and together. In fact, during gait, half of the spine rotates one way following the direction the pelvis is rotating, while the other half of the spine rotates the other way, following the direction of the arm that's swinging back. Sometimes, the spine rotates better to one direction, which creates a habit of rotating to one side more frequently or keeping one foot in contact with the ground more often than the other. The goal isn't to make people symmetrical. Rather, it's to improve proprioception, balance, and connection between the two sides of the body.

Chapter 7

Case study

A few years ago, I began working with Jess who was referred to me with chronic low back pain. As I watched her move, I noticed she was heavy on the right side. She laterally flexed the right spine when she did basic movements. She didn't laterally flex to the left at all. There was very little rotation in her thoracic spine, which meant she wasn't dispersing load well throughout the torso.

I learned through chatting with her that she had been in a car accident where the right side of the car was struck. She was a teenager at the time, and didn't think anything of it. Though she was probably sore for a few days, she didn't consider the impact anything that would have long-term affects. (She has had chronic low back pain since she was in college.)

During a perceived threat, we evolved to fight, flee, or freeze. The freeze response, also known as tonic immobility, is sort of like playing dead. In the face of a life or death situation, sometimes freezing is the best chance for survival (Schmidt et al. 2008). This form of the freeze response results in bradycardia and immobility.

We also freeze when we are assessing a situation. It has been suggested that it's an active way to cope with stress, giving the organism time to anticipate and prepare for an opportunity to counter-attack (Ly et al. 2017).

In humans, when we experience something traumatic like a car accident, sexual assault, child abuse, or combat situations, we aren't always given the opportunity to counter-attack or escape. Sometimes, we are forced to remain still, strapped in ambulance gurneys or immobile under the weight of an attacker, feeling unable to move, even when the threat is gone.

Over the years I have worked with a handful of individuals who appear stuck in a specific holding pattern, hypertonic

in a certain area. I have learned the solution isn't to force a new position on to them; rather, I use gentle coaxing, alternating between gradually exposing the person to new positions and letting the individual be in the position that is comfortable while creating a dialog that focuses attention around how they are moving.

Research supports the role of mind–body practices in individuals with post-traumatic stress disorder (PTSD) (Kim et al. 2013). Both dissociation and depersonalization are commonly associated with PTSD. Dissociation means to lack connections; in a movement setting, dissociation can be thought of as lacking connection with the self, making it difficult to focus attention. Depersonalization is being detached from the body; if I were to say, "My body doesn't feel like it belongs to me," that would be characteristic of depersonalization (Boyd et al. 2018). Slowing down, focusing attention, and inviting self-reflection are all ways to improve interoception, kinesthesia, and proprioception. These improvements, in turn, improve neuroception.

Jess often used words like "heavy" and "pressing down" to describe the sensation of the right side of her back and pelvis. She said the left side felt "light" and "not connected." I explained I wanted her to feel heavier in the left side and to have more connection with her left leg and the left side of her pelvis. She listened, curious, and said, "Wow, I always assumed I just needed to make my right side feel light like my left side. But that isn't it. It's about creating balance."

Over time, she became aware of her tendency to shift over to the right side, particularly when life was stressful. It's well documented that chronic pain is more than just a mechanical issue of a certain muscle being tight, or certain areas needing strengthening. Depression and anxiety are both associated with low back pain. Recognizing if the back feels worse during periods of stress can provide information about a student's physical responses to emotional states (Mirzamani et al. 2005).

She also became stronger. It's important not only to recognize patterns and create opportunities to move differently when there is pain, but to develop opportunities to feel strong and capable. Feeling strong increases self-confidence, and self-confidence makes obstacles in life feel more manageable.

Exercise

Supine rolling, non-segmented

Lie on your back with the knees bent and the feet flat. Pick the right foot up so the knee is bent and the right knee is directly over the right hip. Leave the right leg up as you pick the left foot up so it's in the same position, directly over the left hip.

Make fists with the hands and place the fists between the knees. The knees will gently squeeze the hands (Figure 7.4).

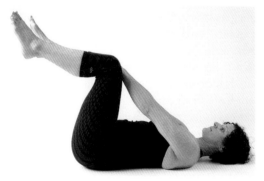

Figure 7.4

Roll to the right, so the left shoulder and left hip come off of the floor. Roll to the left, so the right shoulder and right hip come off of the floor.

Go back and forth between the two positions four to six times. Lower the feet to the floor and rest (Figure 7.5).

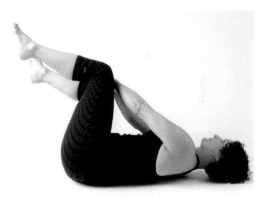

Figure 7.5

Now, pick the right foot up with your knee bent. Angle the right knee out to the right, so it's a little wider than the right hip. The right shin will angle in, making half of a diamond shape.

Do the same thing with the left leg. The feet will be angled in toward each other, almost touching, with the feet relaxed (toes not pointed or flexed). The knees angle out, away from each other.

Place the hands on the outside of the knees so the hands are pressing into the knees and the knees are pressing into the hands. Lift the right shoulder and right hip off the floor, rolling to the left. Return to center and lift the left shoulder and left hip off the floor, rolling to the right. Go back and forth between the two positions four to six times. Lower the feet to the floor and take a moment to breathe and feel the weight of the spine and pelvis against the floor.

Things to consider and observe

When the feet lifted from the ground, did the low back arch away from the floor? If so, cue lifting the feet on the exhale. See if the student can maintain the contact of the ribs against the floor the entire time.

- Was it easier to roll to one side versus the other?

- Did you breathe?

- Which variation was easier – the fists in between the knees, or the hands outside of the knees?

- In the second variation, did the legs stay wide, or did they move toward the midline?

This is an example of a movement that doesn't require a high-threshold strategy to perform. If the student struggles to pick the feet up without arching or rolling the pelvis, working on both motor control exercises and general strength will create the stability required to sustain the supine, bent-knee, hips flexed position while rolling. If the student struggles to roll without falling to one side or is unable to move the spine as a unit, a general strength and motor control program is indicated.

If the student has adequate stability to perform the movement, rolling variations can be implemented as a warm-up or as a standalone core exercise. Rolling challenges the vestibular system, which has a positive effect on balance, and may also down-regulate the sympathetic nervous system, causing a calming effect. It also improves proprioception and kinesthetic awareness.

The spine and hypermobility

Generalized joint hypermobility, which was discussed in Chapter 3, affects 10–20% of the population. It's characterized as hyperextensibility in multiple joints with or without chronic musculoskeletal complaints. Its very close relative, benign joint hypermobility syndrome, is characterized by musculoskeletal pain associated with ligamentous laxity (Kumar & Lenert 2017).

Stability is achieved through both passive and active components. Joint morphology and stiffness of soft tissues structures (such as ligaments) comprise passive mechanisms of stability; muscular strength and neuromuscular properties make up the active mechanisms (Mebes et al. 2008). It should come as no surprise that balance is often reduced in individuals with joint hypermobility, possibly because of the lack of passive stability. This makes active stability in these individuals extra important. Fortunately, active stability can be achieved through neuromuscular exercises, like the rolling exercise above, and general strength.

If you don't have generalized joint hypermobility but you often work with hypermobile students, it's important to remember that exposing students to new positions and movements that require isometric contractions and neuromuscular control around the center of mass will likely create a strong sensation of muscular contraction. While it's true that anyone placed in a new position will feel the sensation of work, remember that in Chapter 3 I said individuals with hypermobility often have heightened interoception. This means their experience of sensation is likely louder than my experience of sensation. From a teaching perspective, being sensitive to their experience is important; so is knowing that the second time they are exposed to the same position, the sensation won't be as loud due to a learning response.

As strength builds, a hypermobile student will become more balanced. Using isometric positions, external load, and exercises that require balance, proprioception, and neuromuscular control are effective ways to help these students feel more stable and connected to their center of mass.

Exercise
Reaching the arms overhead

Lie supine, with the knees bent and the feet flat. Place the right hand on the left ribs. Lift the left arm up in front of you, with the fingertips reaching toward the ceiling and the palm facing across the body. The thumb will be pointing toward the wall behind you (Figure 7.6).

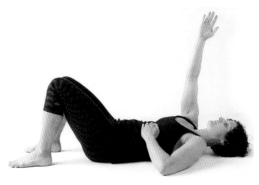

Figure 7.6

As you exhale, reach the left arm back and toward the floor, like it's going over the head. Feel what happens to the ribs beneath the left hand. Inhale and return the left arm to the starting position so it's pointing toward the ceiling.

Repeat this three times, holding the last one for two breaths with the left arm overhead before returning it to the starting position. Switch sides.

Things to consider and observe

What happened to the ribs as the arm reached overhead? If the ribs flared away from the floor, ask the student to use their hand on the ribs to guide the ribs down as the arm reaches overhead and they exhale. What does that feel like?

- Was one side more challenging than the other?

- Did the hand stay in line with the shoulder, or did it move in closer to the head?

- Did the thumb stay pointed at the floor, or did your hand rotate?

This exercise differentiates between shoulder flexion and thoracic extension. If the student's habit is to extend the back to take the arm overhead, this exercise will be surprisingly challenging while the student is learning to differentiate shoulder and back movement. Cueing the breath can help the student feel more clearly how shoulder flexion differs from rib extension. If the hand rotates toward the midline and/or the shoulder moves into internal rotation, causing the thumb to rotate, that can indicate the student has poor kinesthetic awareness of where the arm is in space. This isn't uncommon if the student doesn't have a lot of variability in their arm position throughout the day. Using a prop, like in the variation below, can significantly help with sensing arm position as it moves through space.

Exercise
Dowel variation of reaching the arms overhead

Come into a supine position with the knees bent and the feet flat on the floor. Hold a dowel so the hands face toward the feet. The hands can be shoulder distance apart or wider, depending on shoulder flexibility. Make sure the grip is even across the knuckles and the arms are straight.

As you exhale, keep the arms straight as you reach the arms overhead. Inhale and return your arms to the starting position.

Things to consider and observe

- Does the dowel move backward evenly, or does one side move faster than the other?

- Does the dowel move at an even tempo, or is the movement sped up at any point?

- What happens to the ribs while the dowel moves overhead?

If the student moves one side faster than the other, as long as there is no discomfort, cue the student to see if they can move the dowel evenly overhead. This draws the student's attention to how their arms are moving in relation to each other and often piques their curiosity about the way they are performing the movement. If the student speeds up the tempo of the movement, cue the student to move slowly and with control throughout the motion. For people with a lot of natural shoulder flexibility, there can be a tendency to rush through the section of the motion they are less strong in. Moving slowly requires more muscular effort and may feel like more work than moving slowly.

If this movement is taught with an emphasis on rib awareness and position, it can be a wonderful preparatory exercise before teaching hanging skills or movements where the arms will be placed in an overhead position. Moving on the exhale creates a low-threshold stabilization strategy for shoulder flexion and emphasizes the position of the spine while reaching. It's not that the spine never arches while the arms go overhead, but if that's the student's habit, creating alternative strategies will improve efficiency.

Case study

A client of mine who is in her nineties has struggled off and on with low back pain over the years. She came in recently, frustrated: "Jennifer, I really want to hang, but no one seems to be able to figure out how to let me do it. Can you help me?"

She sits a lot at the bridge table and she tends to look down when she walks. She rarely has an opportunity to lengthen her arms up and away from her spine. I set up a bar that wouldn't move overhead. I had her hold the bar and sit down, so the bar was pulling her arms one way, while gravity pulled her torso the other way. "Ah," she said, "that feels great."

Sometimes, the spine needs traction. Sometimes, the spine needs compression. The best way to create a healthy back is to improve kinesthetic awareness, improve strength, and improve mobility by exposing students to a variety of positions, at a variety of speeds, using a variety of tension.

References

Altun I and Yuksel KZ (2017) Lumbar herniated disc: Spontaneous regression. Korean Journal of Pain 30 (1) 44–50.

Anderson BW and Burns B (2018) Anatomy, thorax, xiphoid process. Treasure Island, FL: Statpearls Publishing.

Berg EJ and Ashurst JV (2018) Anatomy, back, cauda equina, in StatPearls Publishing [Electronic]. Treasure Island, FL: StatPearls Publishing. Available: https://www.ncbi.nlm.nih.gov/books/NBK513251/.

Boyd JE, Lanius RA, and McKinnon MC (2018) Mindfulness-based treatments for post traumatic stress disorder: A review of the treatment literature and neurobiological evidence. Journal of Psychiatry & Neuroscience 43 (1) 7–25.

Bozzao A, Galluci M, Masciocchi C, Aprile I, Barile A, and Passariello R (1992) Lumbar disk herniation: MR imaging assessment of natural history in patients treated without surgery. Radiology 185 (1) 135–141.

Brinjiki W, Luetmer PH, Comstock B, Bresnahan BW, Chen LE, Deyo RA, Halabi S, Turner JA, Avins AL, James K, Wald JT, Kallmes DD, and Jarvik JG

(2014) Systematic literature review of imaging features of spinal degeneration in asymptomatic populations. AJNR American Journal of Neuroradiology 36 (4) 811–816.

Chinn L and Hertel J (2010) Rehabilitation of ankle and foot injuries in athletes. Clinical Sports Medicine 29 (1) 157–167.

Citko A, Gorski S, Marcinowicz L. and Gorska A (2018) Sedentary lifestyle and nonspecific low back pain in medical personnel in north-east Poland. Biomedical Research International, Article ID 1965807.

Cohen R (2001) Interaction of the body, head, and eyes during walking and turning. Experimental Brain Research 136 1–18.

Cramer GD (2014) General characteristics of the spine, in Cramer GD and Darby S (eds) Clinical anatomy of the spine, spinal cord, and ANS, 3rd edn. St. Louis, MO: Mosby.

Dang DC, Dang QK, Chee YJ, and Suh YS (2017) Neck flexion angle estimation during walking. Journal of Sensors, Article ID 2936041.

Davies SJ (2010) "C3, 4, 5 keeps the diaphragm alive." Is phrenic nerve palsy part of the pathophysiological mechanism in strangulation and hanging? Should diaphragm paralysis be excluded in survived cases?: A review of the literature. American Journal of Forensic Medical Pathology 31 (1) 100–102.

Ellenberg MR, Ross ML, Honet JC, Schwartz M, Chodoroff G, and Enochs S (1993) Prospective evaluation of the course of disc herniations in patients with proven radiculopathy. Archives of Physical Medical Rehabiliation 74 (1) 3–8.

Fattahi AS, Maddah G, Motamedikshariati M, and Ghiasi-Moghadam T (2014) Chronic low back due to retroperitoneal cystic lymphangioma. Archives of Bone and Joint Surgery 2 (1) 72–74.

Freburger JK, Holmes GM, Agans RP, Jackman AM, Darter JD, Wallace AS, Castel LD, Kalsbeek WD, and Carey TS (2009) The rising prevalence of chronic low back pain. Archives of Internal Medicine 169 (3) 251–258.

Gizzi L, Rohrle O, Petzke F, and Falla D (2019) People with low back pain show reduced movement complexity during their most active daily tasks. European Journal of Pain 23 (2) 410–418.

Gontijo LB, Pereira PD, Neves CDC, Santos AP, Machado DdC D, and Bastos VHdD (2012) Evaluation of strength and irradiated movement pattern resulting from trunk motions of the proprioceptive neuromuscular facilitation. Rehabilitation Research and Practice, Article ID 281937.

Henmi T, Nakano S, Kanematsu Y, Kajikawa T, Katch S, and Goel VK (2002) Natural history of extruded lumbar intervertebral disc herniation. Journal of Medical Investigation 49 (1–2) 40–43.

Jordan J, Konstantinou K, and O'Dowd J (2009) Herniated lumbar disc. BMJ Clinical Evidence 1,118.

Kawaji Y, Uchiyama S, and Yagi E (2001) Three-dimensional evaluation of lumbar disc hernia and prediction of absorption by enhanced MRI. Journal of Orthopedic Science 6 (6) 498–502.

Kim SH, Schneider SM, Kravitz L, Mermier C, and Burge MR (2013) Mind body practice for posttraumatic stress disorder. Journal of Investigative Medicine 61 (5) 827–834.

Kumar B and Lenert P (2017) Joint hypermobility syndrome: Recognizing a commonly overlooked cause of chronic pain. The American Journal of Medicine 130 (6) 640–647.

Lanser BJ, Wright BL, Orgel KA, Vickery BP, and Fleischer DM (2015) Current options for the treatment of food allergy. Pediatric Clinic of North America 62 (6) 1,531–1,549.

Ly V, Roijendijk L, Hazebroek H, Tonnaer C, and Hagenaars MA (2017) Incident experience predicts freezing-like responses in firefighters. PLoS ONE 12 (10) e0186648.

Mabry LM, Ross MD, and Tonarelli JM (2014) Metastatic cancer mimicking mechanical low back pain: A case report. Journal of Manual & Manipulative Therapy 22 (3) 162–169.

Maslivec A, Bampouras TM, and Dewhurst S (2017) Head flexion and different walking speeds do not affect gait stability in older females. Human Movement Science 55 87–93.

Matijevich ES, Branscombe LM, Scott LR, and Zelik KE (2018) Ground reaction force metrics are not strongly related with tibial bone load when running across speeds and slopes: Implications for science, sport and Wearable tech. PLoS One 14 (1) e0210000.

McGuire JF, Lewin AB, and Storch EA (2014) Enhancing exposure therapy for anxiety disorders, obsessive compulsive disorder, and postraumatic stress disorder. Expert Review of Neurotherapeutics 14 (8) 893–910.

Mebes C, Amstutz A, Luder G, Ziswilier H-R, Stettler M, Villiger PM, and Radlinger L (2008) Isometric rate of force development, maximum voluntary contraction, and balance in women with and without joint hypermobility. Arthritis Care & Research 59 (11) 1,665–1,669.

Menon VK (2019) Mechanically relevant anatomy of the axis vertebra and its relation to hangman's fracture: An illustrated essay. Neurospine 16 (2) 223–230.

Mirzamani SM, Saddi A, Sahral J, and Besharat MA (2005) Anxiety and depression in patients with lower back pain. Psychology Report 96 (3/1) 553–558.

Morasso P, Casadio M, Mohan V, Rea F, and Zenzeri J (2015) Revisiting the body-schema concept in the context of whole-body postural-focal dynamics. Frontiers in Human Neuroscience 9 83.

Mulder T (2007) Motor imagery and action observation: Cognitive tools for rehabilitation. Journal of Neural Transmission 114 (10) 1,265–1,278.

Nijs J, Girbes EL, Lundberg M, Malfiett A, and Sterling M (2014) Exercise therapy for chronic musculoskeletal pain: Innovation by altering pain memories. Manual Therapy 20 (1) 216–220.

Parkhurst TM and Burnett CN (1994) Injury and proprioception in the lower back. Journal of Sport & Physical Therapy 19 (5) 282–295.

Pearce JMS (2004) Sir Charles Scott Sherrington (1857–1952) and the synapse. Journal of Neurology, Neurosurgery & Psychiatry 75 (4) 544.

Purves D, Augustine GJ, Fitzpatrick D, Katz LC, LaMantia A-S, McNamara JO, and Williams SM (eds) (2001) Mechanoreceptors specialized for proprioception, in Neuroscience, 2nd edn. Sunderland, MA: Sinauer Associates. Available: https://www.ncbi. nlm.nih.gov/books/NBK10812/.

Safarini OA and Bordoni B (2019) Anatomy, thorax, ribs. Treasure Island, FL: StatPearls Publishing. Available: https://www.ncbi.nlm.nih.gov/books/NBK538328/.

Scheuer L and Black S (2000) Chapter 7: The thorax, in Scheuer L and Black S (eds) Developmental Juvenile Osteology. Cambridge, MA: Academic Press.

Schmidt NB, Richey JA, Zvolensky MJ, and Maner JK (2008) Exploring human freeze responses to a threat stressor. Journal of Behavior Therapy and Experimental Psychology 39 (3) 292–304.

Sharma V and Kaur J (2017) Effects of core strengthening with pelvic proprioceptive neuromuscular facilitation on trunk, balance, gait, and function in chronic stroke. Journal of Exercise Rehabilitation 13 (2) 200–205.

Steffens D, Hancock MJ, Maher CG, Williams S, Jensen TS, and Latimer J (2014) Does magnetic resonance imaging predict future low back pain? A systematic review. European Journal of Pain 18 (6) 755–765.

Waxenbaum JA and Futterman B (2018) Anatomy, back, thoracic vertebrae. Treasure Island, FL: StatPearls Publishing.

Wong M and Kiel J (2019) Anatomy, abdomen and pelvis, sacroiliac joint. Treasure Island, FL: StatPearls

Publishing. Available: https://www.ncbi.nlm.nih.gov/books/NBK507801/.

Woolf CJ (2011) Central sensitization: Implications for the diagnosis and treatment of pain. Pain 152 (3) 2–15.

Yan YZ, Li QP, Wu CC, Pan XX, Shao ZX, Chen SQ, Wang K, Chen X, and Wang X (2018) Rate of presence of 11 thoracic vertebrae and 6 lumbar vertebrae in asymptomatic Chinese adult volunteers. Journal of Orthopaedic Surgery and Research 13 (1) 124.

Zellmer M, Kemozek TW, Gheidi N, Hove J, and Torry M (2019) Patellar tendon stress between two variations of the forward step lunge. Journal of Health Science 8 (3) 235–241.

Case study

A client was referred to me by his physical therapist for post-rehabilitation on his right shoulder. He had injured it lifting something heavy out of the back of a car and had surgery to repair the injury. Despite following his rehabilitation protocol, he still didn't feel completely confident in the abilities of his right arm. There was a nagging discomfort through the right shoulder area, and a sense of tightness.

As I watched him move, I noticed he was leaning into his right side. His shoulder on the right side was slightly depressed compared to his left shoulder and there was chronic tension in the right upper extremity, like it was bracing for the next traumatic incident.

I cued his attention to his left side, asking him to feel his left arm supporting him in different positions. I introduced shoulder extension, abduction, and external rotation on the right side. I cued in a way that facilitated co-contraction at the shoulder joint, which eliminated discomfort. I taught him how to isolate movement through his scapulae, and we worked on using both hands to grip objects in a variety of ways, focusing on his experience throughout the shoulder girdle.

His discomfort slowly dissipated and as he began to find more confidence and trust that his right shoulder would support him, the hypertonicity through the area decreased. He looked at me one day and said, "It's like my shoulder has PTSD."

Chronic postsurgical pain (CPSP) is a term used to describe chronic pain that lingers for more than three months after surgery. Surgery results in trauma and inflammation from tissues that are cut and handled; this activates nociceptors and can lead to a decrease in nociceptor activation threshold. Basically, the area where the surgery occurred becomes more sensitive, which will change how it's integrated into movement (Reddi & Curran 2014).

Proprioception can also be altered following surgery. Remember that proprioceptors are located in a variety of places throughout the body, including in the skin and extracapsular muscles and ligaments. When there is trauma in these areas because of surgical incisions, the afferent nervous system is impacted, affecting the ability to accurately determine joint position (Jo et al. 2016).

Improving proprioception can be done in a variety of ways. With this client, before I worked on loading the affected shoulder, I began by improving general awareness of the entire upper extremity, specifically, the left arm. Despite the fact that the injury was on the right side of his body, when I observed his movements, he was habitually using his right side more. Giving him movements that required reaching and loading the left arm improved both his kinesthetic awareness and his ability to sense a more accurate location of his center of mass. The heaviness and overuse on the right side was shifting his center of mass to the right; through a combination of foot work, unilateral leg exercises, and rolling movements, slowly he was able to paint a more accurate picture of his body schema and the location of center.

When I finally got to his right shoulder, I worked on a lot more than just the shoulder joint. The shoulder is a complex structure, comprised of several joints that allow rotation to occur. What happens at the shoulder is influenced by the distal portion of the upper limb, aka the hand. The complexity of the upper limb enables it to perform several different movements that require stability throughout the upper extremity.

When you raise an arm, the deep muscles of the torso contract, creating stability throughout the spine. This means any activity that requires movement of the arms also requires a degree of spinal stiffness and stability (Allison et al. 2008). Understanding how the upper extremity works can

continued

help you identify how to create more efficiency and integration throughout the entire structure. To begin, let's look at the hand.

The hand is filled with the ability to gather information, through both touching and grasping objects (Jones 2006). Touching gives you the ability to gather information about the world around you. If you close your eyes and ask someone to place an unidentified object in your left hand, the sensory receptors in the hand will help your mind create a picture about the density, shape, and texture of what you are holding. Your mind will use that information and compare it to previous experience, giving you the ability to make an educated guess about what you are holding.

It's easy to take for granted how sensory rich the hands and fingers are. If the hands are used in repetitive ways to hold or touch predictable objects like keyboards, bags, or phones, they become less adaptable, less mobile, and less informative. The body map of the hands becomes less accurate, affecting everything from the ability to determine miscellaneous objects while blindfolded to the ability of the upper limb to integrate in a wide variety of movements.

Many of the activities of daily life require similar hand and wrist positions. Typing and texting require slight wrist extension and finger flexion. Driving requires slight wrist extension and the fingers flexed, in a loose fist. Few day-to-day activities require the fingers or the wrists to move into full flexion or extension for most people.

In Chapter 2, I gave a practical example of a proprioception exercise involving the hand. If you don't remember doing it, now is a good time to go back and try it. It's an excellent example of how applying force in the form of touch improves kinesthesia, body schema, and ultimately proprioception.

The anatomy of the hand is complex. There are eight small bones in the wrist and 19 bones in the hand (Tang & Varacallo 2018). Like the foot, there are layers of muscles that allow the hand to create several small, finely controlled movements. The complexity of the design allows the hand to hold, throw, and make things (InformedHealth.org 2010; Duncan et al. 2013).

To fully use the hands would require gripping and lifting heavy things, throwing a graspable object, and developing fine motor control by using tools, like crochet needles, a screwdriver, or an instrument. Using the hands in a way that requires integration with the shoulder develops strength; using the hands to make something requires dexterity. Both are important and encouraging students to use the hands in variable ways will enhance efficiency.

Exercise

Making fists and spreading the fingers

Come into a seated position with your arms resting comfortably. Take a moment to feel the arms and hands without looking at them.

How are the hands resting? How are the fingers oriented?

Now, bend the elbows by your sides so the hands are in front of you. Make strong fists, holding for a count of two. Then open the fingers, spreading them wide, holding them for a count of two. Go back and forth between the two positions four times (Figures 8.1 and 8.2).

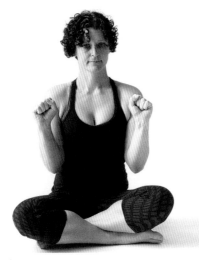

Figure 8.1

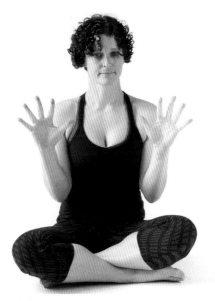

Figure 8.2

Keep the palms open and bring your five fingers together. Spread the five fingers apart. Go back and forth between the positions four times.

Imagine there is glue holding the fourth and fifth fingers together and holding your thumb, index, and third finger together. Separate the third and fourth fingers and then bring them together without letting anything else move. Go back and forth between the two positions four times (the "Spock" for those of you who are *Star Trek* people) (Figure 8.3).

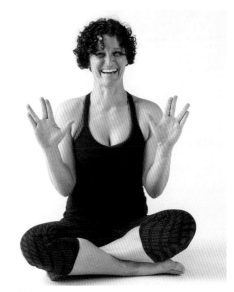

Figure 8.3

Finally, imagine there is glue between the third and the fourth fingers, keeping those two fingers together. Move the index finger and pinky finger away from the third and fourth fingers and then back to the third and fourth fingers. Repeat this four times (Figure 8.4).

Chapter 8

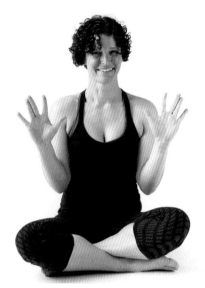

Figure 8.4

When you finish, rest with your hands in a comfortable position. How do the hands feel now?

Things to consider and observe

- Which fingers were hardest to move?

- When you separated the fingers, did they move evenly, or did any of the fingers move more than the others?

- Was one hand more challenging than the other?

- Did you feel echoes of the movement throughout the arm?

- Was it difficult to keep the elbows in?

- Did the jaw clench?

- Did you remember to breathe?

Asking people to isolate movement at the fingers gives you opportunities to assess how they use their hands. I find clients who regularly participate in activities such as putting together furniture, knitting, or playing a musical instrument tend to have a much easier time isolating movement at the fingers than clients who don't participate in these types of activities. Improving individual finger movement can make it easier to cue grip strength, as you will see later.

Maintaining mobility at the fingers and wrist in different positions may also help reduce biomechanical stress on the median nerve. It has been suggested that conditions such as carpal tunnel syndrome occur because of repetitive stress associated with hand and wrist posture and hand force (Loh et al. 2018). Carpal tunnel syndrome is compression of the median nerve at the wrist, causing tingling and numbness in the hand; while there is no sure fire way to prevent anything, there is a possibility incorporating variable hand and wrist movements will lead to more varied use of the hands and wrists throughout the day, lessening the likelihood of repetitive overuse.

Practical application

Before we discuss wrist extension, set a timer for 2 minutes. Move your fingers as many ways as you can think of, moving the fingers individually, together, or sometimes individually and sometimes together. When the timer goes off, take a moment to reflect on your experience.

Taking time to explore is critical for creativity and learning. As a teacher, it's often easy to lose sight of the benefits of small moments of play. As I was rolling on the floor today, with no agenda other than exploration, I found myself wondering, "What if every movement we consider an exercise was actually just a curiosity, a movement someone else thought was interesting enough it should be repeated?" While there are no new movements or exercises, there can be new ways to look at certain skills or movements if you, the practitioner, are willing to take the time occasionally to explore.

I mentioned earlier that everyday life doesn't often require full wrist extension, so it should come as no surprise that many people lack adequate wrist extension and/or hand strength to support themselves in a quadruped (hands-and-knees) position. If the heel of the palm is unable to come into contact with ground when the arm is under the shoulder, it's analogous to the heel of the foot not connecting with the ground – it decreases stability and reduces afferent feedback to the sensory nervous system.

Additionally, the fingers help you feel the ground. Placing weight evenly across the fingers in a hands-and-knees position provide information regarding the density of the surface and, along with the proprioceptors in the wrist, assist with maintaining balance.

If students struggle with mobility in their wrists, it's important to give them stepping stones to begin gently loading the wrists so they can gain strength and mobility. Changing the angle of the torso so that there is less load on the hands and wrists provides students with an opportunity to begin feeling what it's like to have weight in the hands, working on wrist extension in a progressive way. One way to do this is to use a wall, as you will see in the exercise below.

Exercise

Rotating the elbows to feel the pressure on the heel of the palm

Stand facing a wall with your hands on the wall, fingers pointing toward the ceiling. The hands should be in line with the shoulders and the elbows should be straight. Feel the connection of the hands against the wall. Pay attention to the sensation of the heel of the palm against the wall, observing where the weight is located in each hand.

Keeping the arms straight, rotate the elbows in and out a few times. As you do this, observe how the weight changes in the hands. When the elbows rotate in, does the weight go to the outside or the inside of the hands? What does the weight do when the elbows rotate out (Figures 8.5 and 8.6)?

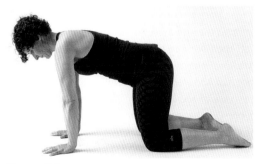

Figure 8.5

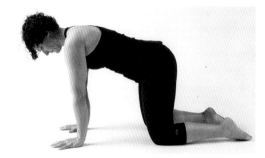

Figure 8.6

Things to consider and observe

- Is the heel of the palm against the wall, or does it lift?

- Do the elbows stay extended as the elbows rotate in and out or do they bend?

- Where is the head in relation to the spine?

- Do the index fingers angle in, out, or do they point straight up toward the ceiling?

For most people, rotating the elbows out shifts the weight toward the thumb side of the hand, inside fingers, and the inside of the palms. The opposite happens when the elbows rotate inward. The weight shifts toward the fourth and fifth fingers and to the outside of the palms.

If someone struggles to keep the heels of the palms against the wall, this suggests a flexibility restriction in the wrist. If there is any discomfort on the side of the wrist that is bent, this indicates closed angle pain. When there is closed angle pain in any joint, the student should consult with a medical professional for further assessment. If it feels like a deep stretch on the bottom portion of the wrist that isn't bent, then it's more than likely a mobility restriction of some kind. Using a combination of neuromuscular techniques and strengthening techniques will result in improvements in mobility over time if they are performed consistently.

If the elbows bend when the student tries to rotate the elbows in or out, the student doesn't know how to isolate elbow and shoulder movement. An example of one way to teach the student how to rotate the arm without bending the elbow can be found in the next exercise.

Remember, this is just an example. There are an infinite number of ways to teach the same concept.

If the student sets up so the index fingers angle in towards each other, that generally indicates the student has a habit of internal rotation in the upper arm. If the student sets up so the index fingers point away from each other, that indicates a habit of external rotation in the upper arm. Neither of these habits are bad; giving the student alternative ways to position their hands increases movement options, flexibility, and strength.

In a quadruped position, to maximize efficiency and share the load between the joints of the upper extremity, the above exercise can be used to find the place where the weight feels loaded in the center heel of the palm and evenly across the fingers. When the torso changes position, like during a push-up or crawling movements, the weight across the hand will also change. This is normal, just like your foot changes position as the torso moves over it during the transition from early to late stance in the gait cycle. The goal isn't to insist on a neutral or centered position throughout a movement; however, it is helpful for people to be able to find a place where they feel maximally supported in positions that are often used as a transition, such as the quadruped position.

Once there is clarity in how changing the position of the elbow affects the sensation of load in the wrist, teaching students to feel how the rotation of the upper arm affects load in the wrist and the hand can also be beneficial.

Exercise
Upper arm rotation and lower arm connection

Facing a wall, take the left hand to the wall so the palm is flat and the fingers point up toward the ceiling. Place your right hand on the upper left arm so you can feel how it moves. Rotate the elbow in and out. What happens to the upper arm?

Switch sides, placing the right hand on the wall and the left hand on the right upper arm as you rotate the right elbow in and out. How does that feel? What happens in the right upper arm as the elbow rotates?

Things to consider and observe

- Is the student able to feel the upper arm rotating when the elbow moves?

- Is one direction easier than the other?

- Is one side easier to feel than the other side?

For most people, as the elbow rotates out, the upper arm internally rotates. As the elbow rotates in, the upper arm externally rotates. Often, due to the natural asymmetries in the body and movement habits, one side is clearer than the other, meaning the student is better able to feel and control the movement in one arm versus the other arm. As the student uses the less clear arm more and pays attention to the sensations they feel while using that arm, awareness and connection improve.

Internal and external rotation of the upper arm happens at the glenohumeral joint, which comprises the glenoid cavity of the scapula and the head of the humerus. This is often what's thought of as the shoulder joint, though as you will discover in a moment, three other joints contribute to the large range of motion available in the upper extremity. The glenohumeral joint is a ball-and-socket joint and is the most mobile joint in the human body due to the shallowness of the joint and the looseness of the joint capsule. It's also the most dislocated joint in the human body (Chang & Varacallo 2019).

Understanding how the movement of the upper arm influences weight in the wrist can make it easier to find subtle weight shifts in positions where weight is placed in the hands. During dynamic movements such as crawling, the upper arm moves into both internal and external rotation as the arm passes under the body and prepares to lift off the floor and move forward, much like the femur moves into internal rotation as the torso passes over the stance foot and into external rotation as the foot prepares to push off of the ground. Just like the foot has muscles that prevent the arch from collapsing as it's loaded, the hand and wrist have muscles that prevent the inner part of the hand from collapsing into the floor during load-bearing activities.

The reverse is also true. If the wrist, elbow, and shoulder lack the flexibility needed to allow the inside of the wrist and thumb to stay in contact with the floor, the base of support to bear load on it decreases. This reduces stability and changes how load is dispersed through the upper extremity. Since proprioception and neuroception are partially dependent on joint mobility and control, it's important to understand how movement at one joint affects movement at the joint above or below it so that support for dynamic movement can be maximized.

Once the student understands the fundamentals of how the upper body supports load using a wall and has adequate mobility and strength in the wrist, the student can begin to incorporate positions that require more wrist loading. This can be done on an elevated surface, such as a plyo box, Pilates table, or yoga blocks using a piked body position or a straight body position. Positions such as down dog can also be introduced; due to the angle of the body relative to the floor, there is less load on the wrists in this position than in a straight-arm plank, which makes it a good progression for wrist loading. Using single-arm down dog positions and traveling down dog positions can further develop strength and mobility in the wrist while integrating dynamic coordination of the glenohumeral joint.

Grip strength

Learning how to flex the fingers is just as important as learning how to extend and spread the fingers. Grip strength utilizes a flexed finger position to hold on and form a seal around the object. It's also an indicator of quality of life and physical well-being as you age (Musalek & Kirchengast 2017). Researchers suggest the strength in the hands indicates general strength and functional ability for activities of daily living. It's also correlated to the likelihood of a cardiovascular event – another way to look at this is the stronger the hands are, the less likely you are to have a heart attack (Leong et al. 2015).

Since everything is connected, it shouldn't be terribly surprising that grip strength is an indicator of hand strength, upper body strength, and heart health. However, despite the importance of grip strength, everyday life doesn't require most of us to hold things tightly on a regular basis. As a result, the connection with how to grip something so the entire arm is involved, not just the fingers, is lost, making it difficult to open water bottles and gas caps or hold heavy objects for long periods of time.

Resistance training, which is defined as using resistance to cause muscular contraction with the intention of building strength, is an effective intervention for anxiety. Most resistance training programs require using external load of some kind to overload the musculoskeletal system and induce a training effect (that is, the person gets stronger). Holding weighted objects of varying sizes is a way to train grip strength.

When you don't feel strong enough to open a water bottle, it can cause anxiety over the ability to do daily tasks, just like not feeling sure footed can cause anxiety and lack of confidence in the ability to navigate the world. A 2017 meta-analysis assessed 16 articles involving more than 900 participants on the effects of resistance training on anxiety outcomes. The results were overwhelmingly positive, leading the authors to conclude resistance training significantly improves anxiety symptoms in healthy participants and those with a physical or mental illness (Gordon et al. 2017). Feeling physically strong translates into feeling mentally strong.

The exercises above explored how load dispersal in the hand affected the feeling of support through the upper torso. When the weight is centered in the heel of the palm with the weight even across the fingers, this generally causes the sensation of work throughout the entire arm. Finding a way to grip objects so the load is dispersed evenly across the hand creates the sensation of work throughout the arm and into the shoulder. Another term for the activation of several muscles around a joint is co-contraction.

Co-contraction is defined as the simultaneous activation of antagonist muscles around a joint. An antagonist muscle is an oppositional muscle. The antagonist to the biceps is the triceps. Dynamic movement requires muscles to work together, providing support and stability to the structure so load can be dispersed up or down the skeleton. In the shoulder joint, co-contraction can be thought of as the contraction of both the internal and external muscles of the rotator cuff to create a sense of stability for the large degree of mobility inherent in the joint.

Co-contraction reduces the effects of perturbation, which makes it easier to maintain balance. Studies suggest co-contraction increases with movement velocity and decreases gradually while learning a novel motor task (Gribble et al. 2003).

Remember Sherrington's law of irradiation in Chapter 7 and how it can be used to teach core stiffness or stability? As the student learns and becomes more efficient at differentiating hip or shoulder movement from torso movement, less effort will be required and conscious irradiation will no longer be necessary. Irradiation can be thought of as a total body co-contraction.

The same is true for any motor task. When someone is asked to perform a familiar task in a new way, there is initially a high sensation of work, as the muscles co-contract and the neuromuscular system determines the amount of muscular effort that is needed to perform the task in this new way. As the neuromuscular system becomes more efficient, less co-contraction is necessary, but stability is still maintained. Muscles get stronger, joints work together more efficiently, and the degree of muscular contraction needed to perform the task is dialed down. This can happen over the course of weeks or it can happen over the course of 5 minutes (if it happens within 5 minutes, the muscles haven't become physically stronger, the neuromuscular system has streamlined the amount of force needed to complete the task). Since the end goal for any task is to perform it in as efficient a manner as possible, it's unnecessary for a student to feel a large degree of co-contraction every time they perform the same task, for months on end. As the student becomes stronger and more coordinated, introducing variation, in terms of load, speed, or position, will create the necessary stimulus to challenge the student.

Exercise

Making fists and connecting to the shoulder

Come into a seated position with the arms straight, the hands resting by your sides, and the palms facing the body, toward each other. Make strong fists with your hands and pretend you are holding something really heavy. Which parts of your fingers do you feel tensing the most?

Now, begin really clenching the middle, ring, and pinky fingers. The thumb and index finger are still engaged, too, but the other three fingers are really working. Does that change the sensation through your arm?

Things to consider and observe

- Did the jaw clench?

- Did the shoulders internally (or externally) rotate? Or was the student able to isolate the initial movement to the hand?

- Did the student remember to breathe?

It's not uncommon for students to struggle with differentiating between hand, shoulder, and jaw movement. It's also not uncommon for students to find it difficult to generate force using their hands in a straight-arm position, but easy to generate force in a bent-arm position, or vice versa. The more joints the student needs to organize, the more challenging the movement becomes because there are more degrees of freedom to keep in check. The exercise below will explore a similar concept (grip) with the arms in a different, and some may say easier, position.

The straight-arm carry position is a movement performed regularly in everyday life. If a student's habit is to carry a bag of groceries by using force generated mostly from the thumb and first finger, the muscles of the arm, specifically the triceps and the external rotators of the shoulder, won't kick in to co-contract and support the movement. The more of the hand you use to grip, the more muscles are used to keep the arm stable (Sathya et al. 2016).

Does this mean you should have students grasp a 2 kg (5 lb) weight while generating as much force as possible across the five fingers of the hand? Only if you are using it to illustrate how much force the student is capable of generating; otherwise, there is no reason to use excessive force while gripping a light object. One of the benefits of using a variety of tools and positions is that the neuromuscular system becomes adaptive and flexible, able to generate the appropriate amount of force necessary for the task.

Exercise
Bent-arm grip using a ball

Place a small ball about the size of a tennis ball in the palm of the right hand; if you don't have a ball, use a rolled up towel that fits in the palm of the hand. Bend the elbow and turn the palm up toward the ceiling. Squeeze the ball, hold for a count of two, and then relax your grip. Do this 10–12 times.

As you squeeze, see if you can begin to feel where the squeezing comes from. You can even place the left hand on the front of the right biceps to feel the biceps muscle contracting when you squeeze and relaxing when the grip relaxes. Eventually, you may even feel the muscles all of the way up into the shoulder contracting and relaxing (Figure 8.7).

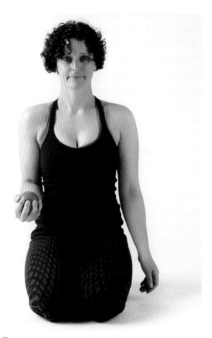

Figure 8.7

After you have finished with the right hand, switch hands. When you have finished both hands, set the ball down and shake out the arms.

Things to consider and observe

- Did the hand stay supinated (palm up toward the ceiling) the entire time?

- Was the student able to initiate grasping the ball with different parts of the hand?

- Did the student remember to breathe?

- How far up the arm did the contraction go?

The supinated grip can be challenging, especially if you are working with someone who spends a lot of time in front of a computer. This particular exercise can be used as a way to assess whether the student feels comfortable with their hands in a supinated position – if they don't, the palm will begin to rotate so it no longer faces up toward the ceiling.

The inability to grasp the ball using different parts of the hand and/or the inability to feel the contraction in the upper arm can be interesting to note. Sometimes, the act of getting stronger enables the student to feel the contraction all of the way up the arm; sometimes, spending more time cultivating the connection between a student's grip and their shoulder gives the student more variability and reduces risk for repetitive use injuries, as you will see in the case study below.

The bent-arm grip exercise using a ball can be performed in a variety of positions, such as with the palm pronated (facing down) or with the palm facing toward the body. It's always interesting to see how small changes impact the ability to feel certain actions; if you perform alternative variations such as these, you may also find the student has a better connection with grasping the ball and co-contraction in the shoulder when they return to the supinated grip. That's the beauty of learning. Sometimes, trying a position that's different or harder makes the initial task easier or clearer.

Chapter 8

Case study

A long-time client went skiing for the first time in several years a few winters ago. He was never a very good skier, and he's also tall, so the goal of the day became to avoid falling by gripping the poles hard for balance.

After a day and a half of skiing, he noticed his right elbow was quite sore. He had essentially given himself tennis elbow, or inflammation of the extensor tendons of the forearm, by gripping harder, and for longer, than he normally does.

(Random fact: Tennis elbow is specific to inflammation on the outside, or lateral, portion of the elbow and forearm. It was originally coined "lawn tennis elbow" in 1882. Golfer's elbow is specific to inflammation on the inside, or medial, portion of the elbow and forearm. Lateral epicondylitis is seven to ten times more frequent than medial epicondylitis, but both commonly occur in people in their forties and fifties (Walz et al. 2010).)

Often overuse injuries are just that: caused from overuse, or overloading tissues before they have a chance to adapt to the new stimulus. It's entirely possible that had he skied two runs, called it quits for the day, and skied two more runs the next day, he would have been fine. It's easy for adults to forget that adaptation occurs during the in-between times, during the rest between attempts. Coincidentally, this is also when learning occurs. The brain and the body require time to process the experience and adapt, whether it's neurologically or physiologically, in order to be more effective and consistent during task performance.

When he came in to see me after his ski trip, I taught him how to grip with his entire upper extremity. It took a couple of sessions for him to internalize how the arm and shoulder supported the gripping action, and it took a couple of months for the sensation of discomfort in his elbow to completely disappear, but he promised me the next time he decides to try skiing, he will do a little less and pay attention to how hard he grips the poles. The more the load is shared in the arm, the less hard just one area needs to work.

A well-coordinated upper extremity is not just the ability to feel the center heel of the palm or the ability to grasp objects. Understanding how to isolate and create movement at the wrist joint is one way to ensure coordinated, efficient movement throughout the hand, elbow, and shoulder.

The wrist moves the hand. Like the ankle, which is also a mobile, complex joint, the wrist can move in several directions. Wrist extension is what the wrist does when the fingers move away from the body. Wrist flexion occurs when the fingers move toward the body.

The wrist can also move laterally (side-to-side), and in a circular motion. The wrist joint, or radiocarpal joint, is a modified ball-and-socket joint. The structure of the wrist allows for the mobility to perform daily function while maintaining an inherent level of stability.

The joint is comprised of the distal radius and three bones of the hand: the scaphoid, lunate, and triquetrum. The stability of the joint is supported by four ligaments that also allow the hand and forearm to rotate together during forearm supination. (Supination occurs when you rotate the palm up toward the ceiling. Pronation is the rotation of the palm toward the floor (Erwin & Varacallo 2018).)

Exercise
Isolating wrist mobility

Bend the right elbow so it's by your side with the palm facing toward the floor in a pronated position. Make a loose fist with the right hand. Move the knuckles up toward the ceiling. Move the knuckles away from the ceiling. Do this four times and switch sides (Figures 8.8 and 8.9).

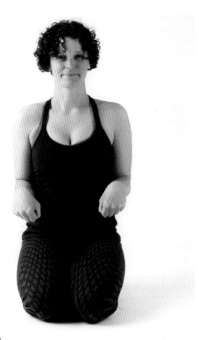

Figure 8.8

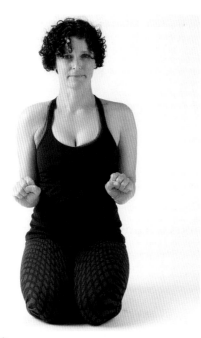

Figure 8.9

Return to the right side, with the elbow bent by your side and making a loose fist with your right hand. Move the knuckles toward your body and away from your body. Do this four times and switch sides.

Finally, with right elbow bent by your side and making a loose fist with the right hand, keep the knuckles oriented toward the ceiling and make a circle with the knuckles. Go four times in one direction and then reverse the direction of the circle and go four times in the other direction. When you finish, switch sides. After you have completed both sides, shake your arms out.

Things to consider and observe

- Which motions were easier to perform? Which were more challenging?

- Was one wrist more coordinated than the other? Was one wrist more stiff?

- Did the knuckles stay oriented toward the ceiling while making wrist circles or did they rotate out?

- Did the jaw clench?

- Did the student remember to breathe?

- Did the elbow remain by the side of the body or did it move away from the body?

Learning to identify which aspects of mobility are challenging helps you create a plan that specifically targets where the student struggles. Often, it's difficult for people to keep the knuckles oriented up toward the ceiling because they couple forearm supination and pronation (which occur at the elbow joint) with wrist abduction and adduction. Learning to isolate the two movements offers more options for movement in the upper extremity. As I have noted previously, when students struggle to perform isolated movements in the upper extremity, either because they lack the strength and mobility or because they don't understand how to do the movement, the muscles in the jaw and neck will tense. Whenever you are watching someone move, occasionally let your eyes observe the person in their entirety instead of fixating on the area performing the movement. Observation can be a powerful tool for understanding a student's movement strategy.

There are two main ways to improve joint mobility. You can ask someone to consciously move a body part around a joint, which is an example of what you just did. The hand moved around the wrist; in order to perform this, the student had to figure out how to make the closed hand move based on information it received on joint angle, tension, and other information it was fed from the mechanoreceptors. This is an example of open-chain mobility (Jewiss et al. 2017).

The other way to work on joint mobility is to anchor a distal body part and move around it. For instance, if you asked the student to imagine their right hand was superglued to a wall or the floor while moving the body around the anchored hand, that would be an example of closed-chain joint mobility.

Life requires both types of mobility, so it's good to incorporate both into a movement practice. Interestingly, sometimes people will have discomfort doing one form of mobility and not have any discomfort doing the other type of mobility, despite the fact both types of mobility require movement around the same joint. The neuromuscular system is funny like that, but what I have learned working with people who have sensitivity is that, if I am creative enough, I can almost always find a way to generate movement at the joint in a pain-free way. To find paths of movement that are pain-free sometimes requires reframing your perspective and thinking outside the box.

Exercise
Wrist mobility in different positions

Face a wall or come into a kneeling position on the floor if it's comfortable. (The kneeling position will result in more weight placed in the hands than facing a wall, so make sure you choose the appropriate starting position for you today.) Place your fingertips on the floor or wall, so the palms of the hands are away from

the surface. Gently, with control, let your hands spread out until the palm comes to the surface, placing as much weight on the hands as you comfortably can (Figure 8.10).

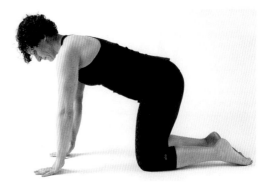

Figure 8.10

Keeping the hands against the wall or floor, shift your weight side to side, forward and backward, diagonally and in a circular fashion. Make the movement small, and if there are areas that feel painful or uncomfortable, don't push into them. Find your edge of comfort and then back off. Spend a minute or two just exploring the different ways you can place pressure on the hands.

Now, walk the hands in different directions. Turn the hands away from each other; turn the hands toward each other; place the backs of the hands against the ground; lift different parts of the hands away from the ground; place fingertips on the ground; and place fists on the ground. Spend 30 seconds to a minute playing with placing the hands in different positions.

Things to consider and observe

- Which positions felt natural?
- Which felt less natural?
- Were there any positions that felt particularly interesting?
- Was there a particular position the student continually returned to?

- Did one hand feel like it had more contact with the floor or wall than the other?

- How did the wrist respond to the different hand positions? Which positions looked particularly strong and stable? Which looked unfamiliar or less coordinated?

This is an example of exploring mobility using both closed- and open-chain mobility work. When the hands remain in contact with the floor and the body moves around them, the student is exploring closed-chain mobility. One of the benefits of repeatedly exposing the joint to different amounts of load at different angles is that it allows the student to spend time in a position that may feel restricted or unusual. The playful approach to the position reduces the sensation of threat generally associated with the position (in this case, a quadruped position), making it more comfortable.

This type of mobility work is also mentally engaging, so it focuses attention and allows the student to move in a way that's less regimented and focused on form or doing things "right." This can be a beneficial way to approach new positions and decrease sympathetic nervous system activity, decreasing neural tone and leading to an increased sense of flexibility.

Additionally, the ability to get off of the floor easily is partially dependent on the ability to load the hands. Most people can regain lost range of motion in the wrist with patience and gradually exposing the hands to the floor in different ways. Rarely is the solution to avoid movement at the joint completely.

Earlier, I mentioned the forearm rotates, allowing the palm to either face forward if the arms are straight, or up to the ceiling if the arms are bent. This motion is called supination and there is actually a muscle in the forearm called the supinator that allows the radius to rotate, which, in turn, moves the hand.

When the forearm rotates the other way, turning the palm so it faces the wall behind you or toward the floor, depending on whether the elbow is extended or flexed, the forearm pronates. There are two muscles, the pronator teres and the pronator quadratus, that pull on the radius, allowing rotation to occur. The names of the muscles that perform these motions aren't important, but it is interesting that the radius is unique in its ability to rotate around the ulna, the other bone of the forearm.

Pronation and supination can occur independently of movement in the upper arm; however, while the humerus doesn't move in an obvious way, supination causes slight external rotation of the humerus and pronation causes slight internal rotation of the humerus (Mansfield & Neumann 2019). In a load-bearing position on the hands and knees, finding the place where the joints stack so the center heel of the palm is roughly under the elbow, which is roughly under the shoulder, is efficient for long periods of load bearing. To maintain this position requires adequate forearm and shoulder mobility so the hand remains pronated while keeping the upper arm in a "neutral" position (that is, not overly internally or externally rotated).

Before we look more intimately at the complexities of the shoulder, try this: bend the left arm so the left elbow is by your side and the left palm is facing toward the floor. Place your right fingers on the top of the left shoulder. Rotate the left palm toward the ceiling. Rotate it back down toward the floor. Do this three or four times while you observe what you feel under the right fingers. Can you feel subtle movements through the shoulder?

If you have someone who struggles with understanding how the forearm moves, creating awareness through touch and observation can highlight the way the upper and lower arm work together, even when one area doesn't appear to be moving. Taking a moment to help people feel these types of connections can make more complex movements smoother and more coordinated.

The anatomy of the upper arm

The upper arm consists of a long bone called the humerus. At the end of the elbow are two knobby protuberances called epicondyles. You have one on either side of the humerus.

Chapter 8

There are two bony articulations that occur at the distal portion of the humerus: the ulna and humerus and the radius and humerus (Karbach & Elfar 2017). These articulations make up what is commonly thought of as the elbow joint.

The proximal portion of the humerus meets the scapula, or what is commonly thought of as the shoulder blade, at the glenuhumeral joint, a ball-and-socket joint formed by the shallow cup of the glenoid fossa of the scapula and the rounded head of the humerus bone (Kadi et al. 2017). This is what people often think of when they think of the shoulder joint; however, as I mentioned earlier, the shoulder joint is actually a complex structure comprised of several joints that allow the upper arm to move. Very close to the glenohumeral joint is the acromioclavicular (AC) joint, the meeting place of the shoulder blade and clavicle, aka collar bone (Wong & Kiel 2018). The AC joint provides stability and mobility to the shoulder joint, and is partially responsible for the arm's ability to move multi-directionally.

As the arm moves, both the scapula and clavicle respond by moving. The clavicle attaches to the sternum at the sternoclavicular joint, which means when the arm moves, not only do the scapula and clavicle move, but the sternum moves as well. The degree of movement depends on how much and at which angle the arm moves. Try this: place your left fingers on the top of your sternum, where the right clavicle forms the sternoclavicular joint. Lift your right arm slowly up toward the ceiling. Do you feel any movement under your fingers? At what point do you feel movement under your fingers?

Moving slowly can highlight the connections that exist during movement by giving the student an opportunity to feel what's happening. Finding these connections is a way to enhance interoception; additionally, slowing down and feeling is a useful tool for learning.

The scapulae sit on top of the ribs on the posterior side of the body. In Chapter 5, we covered how the ribs move during breathing. If the ribs lack the ability to expand posteriorly and laterally during the inhale and exhale, there is less surface area for the shoulder blades to glide on. This isn't necessarily bad, but it may limit range of motion at the shoulder.

The place where the scapulae and ribs connect is interesting because it isn't a true joint. The bones don't articulate the same way as they do in a true joint. The scapulae sit on top of the ribs, not in a groove in the ribs, which means there are no ligamentous connections between the scapulae and the thorax. There are 17 muscles that attach at the scapula, providing the necessary stability to allow for controlled scapular movement when the arm moves. Movement of the scapula is influenced by muscle forces and joint reaction forces from the thoracic surface, AC joint, and glenohumeral joint (Seth et al. 2016).

Basically, a lot of things work together to allow the arm to move several directions. The rest of the exercises in this chapter will explore ways to continue feeling how the different areas of the shoulder (that is, clavicle, humerus, scapula, and sternum) contribute to the unique amount of movement that is available in the arm.

Exercise
Initiating rotation with the upper arm

Come into a seated position, either on the floor or in a chair. Take an exhale and relax the ribs and sternum toward the floor.

Reach the arms straight out to the sides, so they make a "t" with the body. Your hands can either be open or in loose fists, whichever position is more comfortable (Figure 8.11).

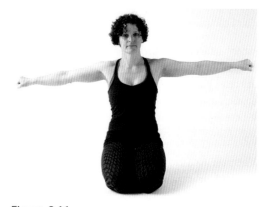

Figure 8.11

Let the bottom of the upper arm rotate forward. What happens to your hands?

Now, let the bottom of the upper arm rotate back. What happens to your hands now (Figure 8.12)?

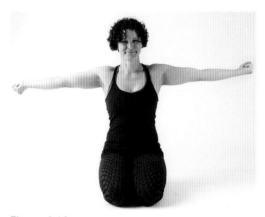

Figure 8.12

Go back and forth between the two movements six to eight times. Allow the motion to be small at first, concentrating on rotating the upper arms internally and externally.

Things to consider and observe

- Where does the movement initiate from?

- Does the hand move first or last?

- Is the student breathing?

- How much of the shoulder girdle is the student allowing to participate in the movement?

The starting position for used for this exercise is called horizontal abduction. It's a challenging position because it involves multiple joints and the orientation of the arms is in the frontal plane instead of the sagittal plane. This tends to be more neurologically complex from a learning perspective.

Subacromial impingement syndrome (SIS) is a common clinical condition affecting 50–86% of people visiting their primary care physician for shoulder pain each year. Its clinical definition is mechanical compression or abrasion of the supraspinatus tendon, subacromial bursa, or long head of the biceps tendon during elevation of the arm. Basically, it hurts to reach the arm overhead or behind the back. There are structural and mechanical changes associated with SIS, such as the compression of the structures in the subacromial space. There are also motor control differences that have been noted in symptomatic versus asymptomatic subjects, specifically reduced upward and external scapular rotation and increased clavicular elevation and retraction (Guitierrez-Espinoza et al. 2019).

Hopefully, it's beginning to make sense that if the scapula and clavicle are unable to move through a full range of motion, there will be a reduction in the arm's capacity to move in an efficient way. It's impossible to know whether specific movement patterns or reductions in range of motion contribute to the presence of pain, but maintaining an efficient shoulder joint that allows the arm to move many different ways involves using the arm in a wide variety of positions. The above exercise can be used to teach movement initiation at the shoulder joint; it can also be used as a warm-up before overhead movements or movements where the arm reaches behind the body. Giving smaller motor control exercises that require focused attention and invite self-inquiry often makes the larger, more dynamic exercises smoother and more coordinated. It's impossible to eliminate injury risk, but asking people to move in a variety of planes, in a variety of ways, keeps the joints – and the mind – healthy.

Case study

A client of mine came in with left shoulder pain. The pain had been intermittent, so she hadn't mentioned it until it settled in and stayed a while. She had a tendency to sleep on her left side, with her shoulder shrugged up and underneath her. She noticed it mostly at night, and occasionally when she reached her left arm behind her.

I turned a kettlebell upside down and had her hold the handles while she performed a squat. "That feels great," she said. "I should walk around holding something like this while it's bothering me."

I chose this kettlebell position, commonly referred to as a "bottoms up" position, because it places the humerus in an externally rotated position and requires co-contraction of the rotator cuff muscles to stabilize the weight. When she

gestured toward where she was feeling irritation, it was in the anterior portion of the left shoulder; choosing a movement that required co-contraction of the shoulder muscles gave her temporary pain relief and reminded her that her shoulder was still functional. It wasn't bad or broken. It could still hold weight and be strong and stable. There were other things that I needed to address, such as teaching her left arm to move into shoulder extension in a pain-free way and improving her scapular mobility, but giving her temporary pain relief and a glimmer of hope was a good place to start.

Remember earlier in the chapter when I asked you to reach your arm toward the ceiling while feeling how the clavicle moved? Let's return to that idea by exploring what it feels like to reach in different planes.

Exercise
Integrating the clavicle with the arm

Place your right fingers on your left collarbone. Reach the left arm in different directions, forward, behind you, above you, in front of you, out to the side, and across you. Spend about 30–45 seconds, reaching the arm and feeling what happens under your fingers (Figures 8.13–8.16).

Once you have finished, switch sides, doing the same thing with the fingers of your left hand on your right collarbone.

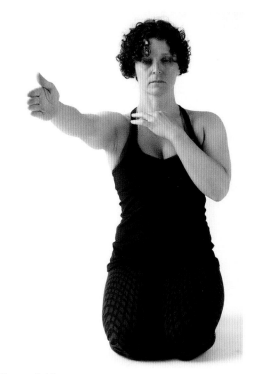

Figure 8.13

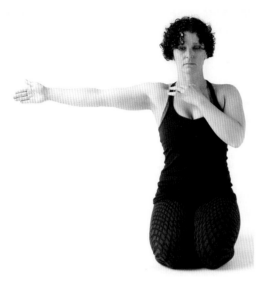

Figure 8.14

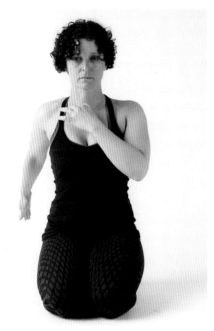

Figure 8.15

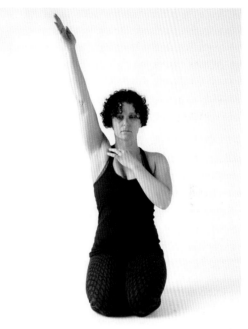

Figure 8.16

Things to consider and observe

- Could you feel the collarbone moving underneath the fingertips when you reached the arm?

- Was one side more "clear" than the other, meaning the movement was more evident?

- Did the student remember to breathe?

Reaching is a great way to teach shoulder integration and improve shoulder mobility. It's a movement that most people deem as safe, and when you ask people to move in multiple directions, they will generally default to the positions that are most comfortable, either because they are the most familiar or they cause the least amount of discomfort. If you notice the student is using the same patterns repeatedly, you can perform the same exercise by asking the student to reach their hand toward your hand.

You can use the information you know about the student's habits to gently challenge the student to move into their blind spots, whether that's behind them, across, up, or down. What's interesting about performing the exercise this way is the student will be focused on something external (your hand), while still creating an internal awareness of the collarbone's movement.

Since the clavicle connects to the scapula at the acromioclavicular joint, it should make sense that the clavicle and the scapula support the arm reaching through integrated movement. When the arm reaches forward, the scapula moves forward, protracting, and the collarbone also moves forward. If the scapula moves back, which happens when you reach your arm behind you, the clavicle moves back. The same is true for reaching the arm up and reaching the arm down. The clavicle moves, responding to the trajectory of the arm and the position of the scapula. The plane in which shoulder flexion is performed, for instance, will affect how much the clavicle retracts, though shoulder flexion will cause clavicular elevation regardless of the plane of motion (Ludewig et al. 2009). The clavicle attaches to the sternum, remember, at the sternoclavicular joint, which we explored earlier. As a result, it also moves when the arm moves, though generally not as much – as you move farther away from the body part where movement is initiated, there is less movement. There is still a response, it's just more subtle and requires more focus to feel.

It's time to explore the scapulae, an area people struggle initially to feel. I have been told repeatedly by clients that understanding how this bone moves creates a sense of freedom and, ultimately, strength through the upper body. It just sometimes takes a bit of patience to help people feel and isolate movement through these bones.

Exercise
Supine scapula and arm integration

Lie down on your back, with the knees bent, the feet flat on the floor, and the arms by your side.

Shrug the shoulders up by your ears. Shrug the shoulders down. Do this four times.

Things to consider and observe

- When the student slides the shoulders toward the ears, do the shoulders move toward the ceiling, away from the floor?

- Do the fingers tense or fidget while the shoulders slide up and down?

- Does the head move?

- When you shrug the shoulders up, in what direction do the hands move?

- When you shrug the shoulders down, in what direction do the hands move?

- Can you feel the shoulder blades moving against the floor?

When the shoulders move up, the hands slide up. When the shoulders move down, the hands slide down. When your shoulders move up, the shoulder blades move up. When the shoulders move down, the shoulder blades move down. These areas are all connected.

If someone lacks mobility in the shoulder blades or doesn't understand how to isolate scapular elevation and depression, the shoulders will move forward as the student elevates the shoulders, or other areas, such as the neck or hands, will assist with the movement. The floor provides kinesthetic feedback, allowing the student to feel what their tendencies are and providing a safe environment while exploring scapular elevation and depression. Teaching upper body coordination with lots of tactile feedback initially, such as on the floor, makes it easier to transfer the same concept to positions where there is less tactile feedback. Often, I will use a movement such as this in a warm-up so I can refer back to it when the student is doing something more complex. For instance, if I have the student performing a variation of an L-sit prep, I might cue, "Push the hands into the box. Remember how the hands moved down when your shoulder moved down on the floor? Do the same action here. See if you can feel your shoulder blades moving down as well, just like they did on the floor." The more connections I can help students create, the more the skills and cues that I use make sense and can be easily implemented.

Exercise
Protraction and retraction in quadruped

Come into a quadruped position with the elbows on the floor instead of the hands. Place the elbows under the shoulders and the knees under the hips.

Press the elbows into the ground. Observe what direction the shoulders move and what happens in the shoulder blades (Figure 8.17).

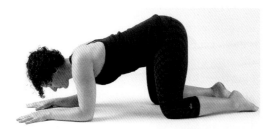

Figure 8.17

Keep the forearms and elbows pressing into the ground and bring the shoulder blades toward each other, retracting them. Maintaining the pressure on the elbows and forearms, continue to press them into the ground as you bring the shoulder blades away from each other, protracting them. Go back and forth between these two positions four to six times (Figure 8.18).

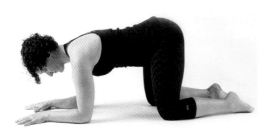

Figure 8.18

Things to consider and observe

- What did the head and eyes do as the shoulder blades moved toward each other and away from each other?

- Was the student able to isolate protraction and retraction, or did the shoulders elevate during the movement?

- Did the student remember to breathe?

This is an example of a closed-chain exercise to teach shoulder blade protraction and retraction. By shortening the lever arm and reducing the degrees of freedom involved, the student has fewer body parts to organize, making the shoulder blade action more obvious. If the person you are working with struggles to isolate movement at the shoulder blades, you may observe the head nodding or shoulder elevation as the student attempts to move the shoulder blades apart and together. You can regress the exercise further by having the student perform the action with the forearms against the wall; you can also progress the exercise by performing the movement in a forearm plank or straight-arm push-up position.

Maintaining the pushing action of the forearms the entire time forces the student to move with control. This translates well to prone pushing movements, such as push-ups and crawling variations. Students who initiate the lowering down action of the push-up by retracting their shoulder blades often lose the pushing action of the hands; when students understand how to continuously push while lowering the body down, the coordination in the scapulae generally improves and the retraction occurs in a more controlled manner.

Exercise
Initiating pulling

For this exercise, you will need a blanket and a surface that isn't sticky, like hardwood or laminate flooring.

Come into a forearm quadruped position, with the elbows on the floor under the shoulders, and the shins and knees on the blanket with the knees under the hips (Figure 8.19).

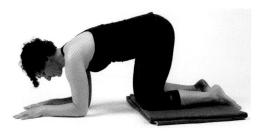

Figure 8.19

Press the elbows into the floor and begin pulling the elbows toward the knees so the knees (and blanket) slide in to meet the elbows. Move the elbows forward and repeat the movement, sliding across the floor four to six times (Figure 8.20).

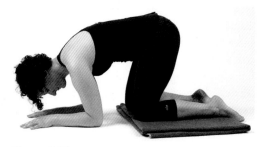

Figure 8.20

After you have finished, come off of the blanket, set yourself up in the same position, and pull the elbows toward the knees, creating the same action in the arms without the knees sliding in. Hold for three or four breaths.

Things to consider and observe

- What happens in the shoulders during pulling?
- What happens in the shoulder blades?
- Where was the head?
- Where did the eyes look?
- Was the student able to mimic the same pulling action without the blanket?

Pulling can be explored several different ways. You can pull something toward you, which is what happens when you ask someone to pull the blanket toward the elbows. You can also use the arms to pull down, which is what happens when you pull the elbows toward the knees without the blanket.

In a movement like a pull-up, you can think of pulling the bar toward the floor, or you can think of pulling the body toward the bar. These two cues will feel different; generally, pulling the bar toward the floor feels like a stronger, more coordinated action, just like pulling the blanket toward the knees usually requires less cueing and is performed in a more intuitive way than statically pulling the elbows toward the knees.

Curiously, learning to generate force while pulling the arms down can sometimes make the movement reaching the arms overhead feel more easeful. You can even turn the isometric action of pulling the elbows toward the knees into a push–pull exercise by having the student pull the forearms toward the knees, bringing the torso forward followed by pushing the forearms into the floor and away from the knees, bringing the torso back toward the hips. Using the forearms to direct movement is a way to use focused attention and force to clarify the actions of the arms and their relationship to the shoulder blades. The movement can be varied by asking the student to perform the movements with their arms offset, so one elbow is forward of the other, or you can have the student place one forearm on the ground and one hand on the ground while performing any of the above variations. Remember, variety enhances understanding.

Exercise
Loading the hands in different positions

Come into a seated position on the floor with your hands behind you, fingers pointed away from you, knees bent and feet flat on the floor.

Begin pressing the hands into the floor. Feel what happens in the shoulder blades (Figure 8.21).

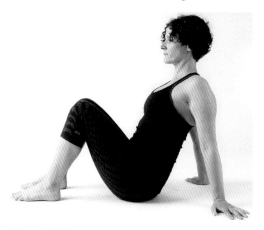

Figure 8.21

Tip your knees to the left, allowing the inside of the left foot and the outside of the right foot to lift as the knees come closer to the ground. As this happens, lift the right hand away from the floor. Keep pressing the left hand into the floor as you come on to your left hip (Figure 8.22).

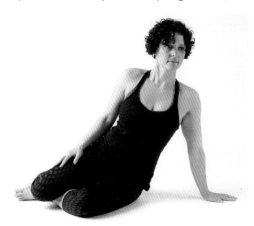

Figure 8.22

Return the knees to the center position and bring the right hand back to the floor, pressing both hands strongly into the ground. Tip the knees to the right, allowing the inside of the right foot and the outside of the left foot to lift away from the ground. The left hand will come away from the ground as you strongly push the right hand into the floor, coming onto your right hip.

Go back and forth between the left and right sides, four to six times. As the hands connect with the floor, press into them strongly.

Things to notice and observe

• Is one side easier to turn to than the other?

• Do both hands press equally into the floor?

• Where is the head?

• Where are the eyes?

Using the hands to support the weight of the body in various positions on the floor is important for getting up off of the ground. This type of exercise also improves neuroception in different floor positions, which is important in the event of a fall. If the student lands in a position that is semi-familiar, the pathway to getting back up will be more obvious.

If the eyes and the head are looking down, there will be less efficiency in the torso. Learning to look out and sense body position improves proprioception, kinesthetic awareness, and body schema.

This same exercise can be performed without cueing the hands. The emphasis, then, becomes one of creating ease and fluidity rather than strength and force. Both are important; both will create connection with the arms in different positions. The question always becomes: what does the student need in this particular moment?

There is a complexity to the upper extremity that is both interesting and unnecessarily mysterious. The hands and their function is easy to gloss over and ignore in movement settings; it's just as easy to become overly fixated on muscular tightness and imbalance in the shoulder girdle. Instead of worrying about what's tight and what's not, watch the student move. Observe the student's habits, assess what positions bring up fear, and find a way to negotiate movement in different positions, slowly and gently at first, progressing to more dynamic movements as the student becomes comfortable. There is no reason people in their seventies can't develop the grip strength and shoulder mobility needed to hang from a bar, support their weight in a straight-arm plank position, or, my current favorite, navigate objects to vault over or get down on the floor.

Hands and arms are used to gesticulate, to create emotion and enhance a story. They interact with tools that interact with the environment, enabling you to type, open doors, and make art. They swing forward and back during gait, creating balanced momentum. Hands gather information about the person you are touching or the object you are grasping. The connection between the hands to the torso gives you stability and strength, but can also give you gentleness and fluidity. Improving awareness of the hands, arm, and shoulders is an opportunity to relate more fully with the world.

References

Allison GT, Morris SL, and Lay B (2008) Feedforward responses of transverses abdominis are directionally specific and act asymmetrically: Implications for core stability theories. Journal of Orthopaedic & Sports Physical Therapy 38 (5) 228–237.

Chang IR and Varacallo M (2019) Anatomy, shoulder and upper limb: Glenohumeral joint. Treasure Island, FL: StatsPearls.

Duncan SFM, Saracevic CE, and Kakinoki R (2013) Biomechanics of the hand. Hand Clinic 29 483–492.

Erwin J and Varacallo M (2018) Anatomy, shoulder and upper limb: Wrist joint. Treasure Island, FL: StatPearls Publishing.

Gordon BR, McDowell CP, Lyons M, and Herring MP (2017) The effects of resistance training on anxiety: A meta-analysis and meta-regression analysis of randomized controlled trials. Sports Medicine 47 (12) 2,521–2,532.

Gribble PL, Mullin LI, Cothros N, and Mattar A (2003) Roles of concentration in arm movement accuracy. Journal of Neurophysiology 89 (5) 2,396–2,405.

Guitierrez-Espinoza H, Araya-Quintanilla F, Zavala-Gonzalez J, Gana-Hervias G, Martinez-Vizcaino V, Alvarez-Bueno C, and Cavero-Redondo I (2019) Rationale and methods of a randomized clinical trial to compare specific exercise programs versus home exercises in patients with subacromial impingement syndrome. Medicine 98 (30) e16139.

InformedHealth.org (2010) How do hands work? [Electronic] Cologne, Germany: Institute for Quality and Efficiency in Health Care (IQWiG).

Jewiss D, Ostman C, and Smart C (2017) Open versus closed kinetic chain exercises following an anterior cruciate ligament reconstruction: A systematic review and meta-analysis. Journal of Sports Medicine 4721548 1–10.

Jo S, Park S-B, Kim MJ, Kim T, Park KI, Sung J, Park UJ, Kim YS, Kang BJ, and Lee KH (2016) Comparison of balance, proprioception and skeletal muscle mass in total hip replacement patients with and without fracture: A pilot study. Annals of Rehabilitation Medicine 40 (6) 1,064–1,070.

Jones EG (2006) The sensory hand. Brain 129 (12) 3,413–3,420.

Kadi R, Milans A, and Shahabpour M (2017) Shoulder anatomy and normal variants. Journal of Belgian Society of Radiology 101 (Suppl 2) 3.

Karbach LE and Elfar J (2017) Elbow instability: Anatomy, biomechanics, diagnostic maneuvers, and testing. Journal of Hand Surgery America 42 (2) 118–126.

Leong DP, Teo KK, Rangarajan S, Lopez-Jaramillo P, Avezum A Jr, Orlandini A, Seron P, Ahmed SH, Rosengren A, Kelishadi R, Rahman O, Swaminathan S, Iqbal R, Gupta R, Lear SA, Oguz A, Yusoff K, Zatonska K, Phil JC, Igumbor E, Mohan V, Anjana RM, Gu H, Li W, and Yusuf S (2015) Prognostic value of grip strength: Findings from the prospective urban rural epidemiology (PURE) study. The Lancet 386 (9,990) 18–24.

Loh PY, Yeoh WL, Nakashima H, and Muraki S (2018) Deformation of the median nerve at different finger postures and wrist angles. PeerJ 6 e5406.

Ludewig PM, Phadke V, Braman JP, Hassett DR, Cleminski CJ, and LaPrade RF (2009) Motion of the shoulder complex during multiplanar humeral elevation. The Journal of Bone & Joint Surgery 91 (2) 378–389.

Mansfield PJ and Neumann DA (2019) Structure and function of the elbow and forearm complex, in Mansfield PJ and Neumann DA (eds) Essentials of kinesiology for the physical therapist assistant, 3rd edn. St. Louis, MO: Mosby.

Musalek C and Kirchengast S (2017) Grip strength as an indicator of health-related quality of life in old age – a pilot study. International Journal of Environmental Research on Public Health 14 (12) 1,447.

Reddi D and Curran N (2014) Chronic pain after surgery: Pathophysiology, risk factors, and prevention. British Medical Journal 90 (1,062) 222–227.

Sathya P, Kadhiravan V, Ramakrishnan KS, and Ghodake AR (2016) Association between hand grip strength and shoulder power in intercollegiate cricket players. International Journal of Innovative Research in Science, Engineering and Technology 5 (3) 3,085–3,091.

Seth A, Matias R, Veloso AP, and Delp SL (2016) A biomechanics model of the scapulothoracic joint to accurately capture scapular kinematics during shoulder movements. PLoS One 11 (1) e0141028.

Tang A and Varacallo M (2018) Anatomy and upper limb, hand carpal bones [Electronic] Treasure Island, FL: StatPearls Publishing.

Walz DM, Newmnam JS, Konin GP, and Ross G (2010) Epicondylitis: Pathogenesis, imaging, and treatment. RadioGraphics 30 (1) E125–E147.

Wong M and Kiel J (2018) Anatomy, shoulder and upper limb: Acromioclavicular joint. Treasure Island, FL: StatPearls Publishing.

The pelvis

Case study

A client came in recently with discomfort radiating up her neck and down into her chest. It was muscular tightness accompanied by a dull ache that was primarily on her right side, though the left side was experiencing similar sensations to a lesser degree. It was uncomfortable to lift her arms and she was unable to bear weight on her arms, regardless of the position. I tried having her place her hands against the wall, but even with the support of the wall, the position caused too much discomfort for her to remain there for any length of time.

I could tell by the way she was moving she needed to feel her left abdominals, and there was something missing with the way she was coordinating her left leg into movement. I wasn't sure what it was, but as I began having her move gently in positions that were pain free, I began to wonder if helping her feel the left side of her pelvis would help.

I had her come into a seated position on a plyo box so her feet were flat on the floor with a yoga block against the box and behind her left heel. "Pull your left heel into the block and breathe four times," I instructed.

In one of those magical movements that happen every once in a while, I watched as her body completely re-organized itself. "Wow," she said after the fourth breath. "That seems like such a simple thing, but I just felt everything up here release," she said, gesturing toward her neck and chest.

When she stood up, her shoulders, which had been visibly uneven when she walked in, were level and she was standing in a more balanced way in her feet. We did it one more time, just so she could remember how to do it, and I told her to do it once a day until I saw her next, which was four days later. "The sense of things adjusting will become less and less," I said.

What happened? Why did pulling a heel into a yoga block work? It's impossible to know for sure – perhaps it was just the right stimulus at the right time, but consider that the pelvis is made up of two halves located just below the center of mass. Subtly changing the position of one of the halves will change how the spine organizes above the pelvis. Changing the position of one area, in this case the pelvis, affects the organization of the spine and femur. Additionally, by having her pull back, it enabled her to feel her left hamstring, which originates at the left ischial tuberosity of the pelvis. The ability to feel force improved proprioception and body schema, so not only was there a physical change in position, there was a neuromuscular change in experience. The pelvis, as you will see throughout this chapter, plays an important role in gait. The muscles that comprise the pelvic floor respond to the breath, mirroring the up and down movement of the diaphragm with each inhale and exhale, and its proximity to the center of mass means its position can have a profound impact on both the spine and the lower extremity.

The pelvis is the attachment point for several muscles that make movement at the hip possible. There are several muscles at the base of the pelvis that support the pelvic organs. The pelvis creates power, generating forward propulsion during throwing and dissipating load from the lower extremity to the upper extremity during running and walking.

Chapter 9

Pelvis: structure

The sacrum meets the fifth vertebrae of the lumbar spine at the lumbosacral joint. The sacrum, a triangular shaped structure comprised of five fused vertebrae, connects to the pelvis at the ilium bones at the sacroiliac joint. This means each person has two sacroiliac joints (SI joints), one on the right and one on the left. Strong ligaments support the joint, providing sufficient flexibility for the transfer of force to and from the lower extremities and the lumbar spine (Vleeming et al. 2012). The ligamentous support makes the sacroiliac joint a stable structure that isn't prone to dislocating or slipping. While it's estimated that 10–30% of low back pain cases are attributed to SI joints, evidence for the SI joint as a causative contributor to low back pain is very limited (Booth & Morris 2019).

Not only is the SI joint anatomically stable because of its shape and structure, it also benefits from something called force closure. Force closure refers to the muscles, fascia, and ligaments that attach to the bony surfaces of the pelvis and provide compressive force to the joint based on position. Another way to think of this is force closure adapts to the SI joint's stability needs based on internal and external demands.

There are three bones that make up the pelvis: the aforementioned ilium, the ischium, and the pubis. There are two sides of the pelvis, and each side of the pelvis consists of one set of these three bones. The place where the three bones of the pelvis intersect is the acetabulum. The head of the femur, the long bone of the leg, fits neatly into the acetabulum, which is cup-like and allows for large degrees of movement because of its structure. The anatomical name for this joint is the acetabulofemoral joint; the common name is the hip joint.

The muscles that make up the floor of the pelvis contract and relax during breathing. They also support the pelvic viscera and resist increases in intra-abdominal pressure (Park & Han 2015). The pelvic floor is innervated by nerves from the sacrum, while the gluteal muscles on the outside of the pelvis are innervated by nerves from L4, L5,

and S1. The superior gluteal nerve and the inferior gluteal nerve provide afferent and efferent feedback for hip rotation and stability.

The tenth cranial nerve is the vagus nerve. Cranial nerves are nerves attached to the brain that are primarily responsible for sensory and motor functions of the head and neck (Hagan et al. 2012). There are 12 pairs of cranial nerves, most of which are considered part of the peripheral nervous system, except for cranial nerves I and II, which are considered part of the central nervous system.

The vagus nerve connects the brain to the abdomen and its tone increases when there is more parasympathetic activity in the nervous system. This results in a slowing of the heart rate and regulated digestion (Breit et al. 2018). Chronic pelvic pain and tightness, an issue affecting anywhere from 6–27% of women worldwide and that is often associated with irritable bowel syndrome, interstitial cystitis, and endometriosis, decreases when the vagus nerve is stimulated (Speer et al. 2016). Research also suggests symptoms related to chronic pelvic pain improve when gentle yoga poses during menses are performed or acupuncture is paired with electrical stimulation (Udoji & Ness 2013). What these things all have in common is they down-regulate sympathetic nervous system activity and increase vagal tone. Another way to look at this is for the pelvis to do its job well, the ability to tap into a state of relaxation occasionally is important. The breathing exercises at the end of Chapter 3 are a great starting place for restorative movement ideas.

There are 25 muscles that cross the external portion of the pelvis, most of which control movement at the hip joint. The more superficial muscles are strong, producing power and generating the force necessary to jump, run, and step up on tall objects. These muscles also allow a diagonal transfer of power from the upper to lower extremity, allowing you to propel an object forward a long distance. The deeper layers of muscle provide stability to the hip joint, much like the rotator cuff muscles of the shoulder provide stability to the glenohumeral joint (Gold & Varacallo 2019).

At the base of the pelvis, each ischium protrudes forming the ischial tuberosities, also known as the sitting bones. The ability to feel them against the surface on which you are sitting provides the neuromuscular system feedback regarding position of the pelvis. The ischial tuberosities are also the attachment points for the hamstring tendons. The hamstring is comprised of three muscles that reach down the back of the leg and is innervated by the sciatic nerve; sciatica, a form of low back pain, is characterized by pain radiating into the hamstring and calf along the course of the sciatic nerve (Juunger et al. 2019).

It's not uncommon for people to spend most of their time sitting on soft surfaces, unable to feel the position of the pelvis or the ischial tuberosities. This isn't necessarily bad, but it can reduce pelvis proprioception. In Chapter 1, you performed a proprioceptive exercise that involved rolling forward and back on the sitting bones, reminding you where the sitting bones were located and providing a reference point for different pelvis positions.

Rolling behind the sitting bones placed the pelvis into a posterior pelvic tilt. Rolling in front of the sitting bones placed the pelvis into an anterior pelvic tilt. Both of these positions are necessary for the functions of everyday life. One is not better than the other.

The ability to control movement at the pelvis creates more options and frees up mobility at the hip joint; if the pelvis stays in one position most of the time, the femur will move in the hip socket, but the hip socket won't move as freely over the femur. Healthy hips are predicated on both the femur moving in the socket and the socket moving over the thigh bone. Remember how we talked about open- and closed-chain mobility in Chapter 8? The same principle applies here. To maximize integrated movement, it's important to utilize both open- and closed-chain mobility at the hip joints.

Pelvis movement also keeps both the internal and external muscles of the pelvis mobile, strong, and healthy. This helps with issues like urinary incontinence and pain during intercourse, and creates a sense of ownership over the entire body.

It's worthwhile to note that trauma can alter movement in the pelvis and hips. I mentioned earlier that some people who have experienced trauma will have a freeze response that lasts long after the trauma has ended. Trauma involving the pelvis can cause the pelvis to appear frozen and rigid, even during activities like walking, where efficiency and coordination depends on the pelvis rotating in a three-dimensional way (Lewis et al. 2017).

I have worked with two different women who labored for long periods of time during the birth of their children, only to be rushed into emergency cesarean sections. One of them lost a significant amount of blood directly after surgery, and both pushed for several hours. These types of events can change people's body schemas, affecting their relationship with the body parts involved and, ultimately, impacting how the body parts are integrated into movement. Part of my work included creating awareness around how to consciously move the pelvis and then helping them coordinate the pelvis into more dynamic movements.

Exercise
Pelvic tilts, back, and hip awareness

Lie down on your back with your knees bent and your feet flat on the floor. Feel the weight of your pelvis against the floor.

Gently roll your pelvis back, taking the arch of your low back closer to the floor. Pause for a second, breathing. Now, gently roll your pelvis forward, arching your low back away from the floor a little bit. Pause for a second, breathing. Go back and forth between these two positions a few times, feeling how rolling the pelvis affects your back.

Now, shift your perspective to the hip joints. Place your fingers in the place where the hip creases in the front of the pelvis and continue making the movement of tilting the pelvis forward, arching your back away from the floor, and back, moving the low back toward the floor. Can you feel the movement beneath the fingers? Can you feel how the pelvis is moving around the thigh bones (Figure 9.1)?

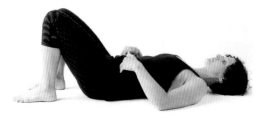

Figure 9.1

Things to consider and observe

- Did the movement appear forced?

- Which direction was easier: anteriorly tilting the pelvis or posteriorly tilting the pelvis?

- Did anything change when the focus shifted to the hip crease?

- Did the student remember to breathe?

If the student struggled to perform the movement in an easy way, suggest making the movement smaller. People who have experienced low back pain are often unclear about how the pelvis moves and how to control pelvic movement. There may be a tendency to overexert by tensing in other parts of the back or body, or by using a high-threshold bracing strategy in the abdominals. Making the movement smaller, or imagining the movement before performing it, can be good ways to teach the student how to perform this movement in a gentle way.

When you lie down on your back with the knees bent and the feet flat, the floor provides information to the afferent nervous system via the pressure it exerts on the body. This helps you feel how the action of the pelvis influences what happens at the spine. Feeling how this movement works on the floor makes it easier to translate the action into other positions such as standing or tall kneeling.

During the swing phase of gait, the leg swings forward, the pelvis moves forward. When the foot lands and is in contact with the floor, the pelvis moves in and over the leg until the foot is beneath it; then it moves out and back (Chan & Rudins 1994).

Each side of the pelvis is referred to as a hemipelvis. The two sides of the pelvis work symbiotically during gait, coordinating with the position of the leg (Musielak et al. 2016).

I mentioned earlier we are all asymmetrical. This can include how the two sides of the pelvis are used. Sometimes, people will favor having one hemipelvis forward and one back. This isn't bad, it's just less efficient than having two sides of the pelvis move in an alternating fashion during the gait cycle.

Exercise
Pelvic rotation awareness

Lie on your back with the knees bent and the feet flat. Place your fingers on the anterior superior iliac spines (ASIS), aka the two front pelvis bones.

Allow the knees to tilt to the right, so the outer edge of the left foot comes away from the floor and the inside edge of the right foot comes away from the floor. Bring the knees back to center and then tilt the knees to the left.

Go back and forth tilting the knees one way and then the other. What's happening beneath your fingers when the knees tilt to the right? What about when they tilt to the left?

Things to consider and observe

- Can you feel the weight of the pelvis rolling against the floor?

- What's happening beneath the fingers as the pelvis rolls?

- Does the tilting of the legs happen in a fluid manner, or does one specific area lead the movement?

- Is one side more easeful than the other?

When the knees tilt right, the pelvis rolls to the right. Since the pelvis is moving, there will be movement under the fingers. When the knees tilt to the left, the pelvis rolls to the left and the sensation under the fingers will change. Connecting students to the rolling sensation of the pelvis on the floor improves kinesthetic awareness and motor control – the ability to feel the movement makes it easier to translate the sense of pelvic rotation in split stance and walking movements.

This exercise is a great cool-down after leg strengthening work. Allowing the pelvis to move in a very safe, relaxing way after long periods in a stable stance and/or generating significant amounts of force acts as a nervous system re-set, down-regulating the sympathetic nervous system. (Rocking in general seems to down-regulate the SNS, which can be useful for individuals who habitually experience high amounts of stress.)

Exercise
Using the feet to generate pelvic rotation

Lie down on the floor with the feet flat and the knees bent. Place the fingers against the ASIS. Reach the right foot into the floor. Relax the pressure of the right foot and reach the left foot into the floor. It's like you are walking, reaching one foot and then the other. Go back and forth, reaching the right and then the left foot, four to six times (Figures 9.2 and 9.3).

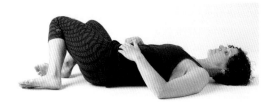

Figure 9.2

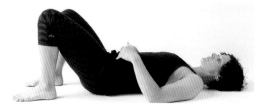

Figure 9.3

Things to consider and observe

- What happens beneath the fingers?
- When the left foot reaches into the floor, does the lift hemipelvis roll to the right? What about when the right foot reaches into the floor?
- Is one side more connected than the other?
- When the right foot reaches into the floor, does the right knee shift forward, responding to the action? What about the left knee when the left foot is reaching?

It can be difficult for people to feel how the action of reaching the foot into the ground causes movement in the pelvis. Teaching students how to feel when the pelvis moves makes it easier to feel when it isn't moving (this same exercise could be taught keeping the pelvis purposefully still; it would feel different, causing the sensation of more muscular work). For students who tend to overwork and use excessive muscular effort to accomplish a task, understanding the connection between the foot and the pelvis can improve efficiency.

As I noted in Chapter 5 while discussing the feet, it can be difficult for people to understand how to push the feet into the ground. The supine, bent-knee position allows the student to focus their attention on pushing the foot without worrying about maintaining balance. This can improve integration by clearly demonstrating how pressing one body part into a fixed object, like the ground, affects the joints up into the torso as it responds to the force generated from the push.

Contextual interference

Performing new movements or making new physical connections can feel frustrating. Students may say things like, "I can't do this," or, "My body doesn't move that way," or, "I'm not built to move like you." Helping students reframe their attitude toward learning new movements is just as important as helping students build strength and mobility. Everyone is capable of learning, regardless of age.

It can be helpful to remind students that practicing and attempting the movements is only one part of the learning process. I discussed self-reflection earlier, which is a form of processing after the practice has taken place. I also mentioned learning happens in the in-between times, during the rest between attempts. I implement this concept frequently with students when I introduce new movements or skills. The first set never goes very well. It's awkward and disjointed as the student attempts to move their body in an unfamiliar way. After a few attempts, I have the person move on to something else that's comfortable and that they know how to perform comfortably.

A few minutes later, I bring the person back to the new exercise. It's always easier. Not perfect, but a little more coordinated and a little more stable feeling if it's a strength-based movement, or a little more supple if it's mobility-based.

If I add the new skill in occasionally, at different times, over the next month, it continues to improve until the person "gets" it. This idea is at odds with human nature – there is an assumption that practicing something, over and over again, exactly the same way each time, will result in steady improvement.

Curiously, that's not how it seems to work. Motor learning research repeatedly demonstrates that contextual interference is an effective way to improve learning retention and skill acquisition (Rad et al. 2012). This means that if someone is struggling with a specific coordination or skill, stepping away from it to practice something else may make the skill feel easier when the student returns to it, especially if the skill is revisited in a slightly different way. The student's ability to move from the cognitive stage to the associative stage of learning is facilitated by not performing the skill repetitiously in the same way.

As I have mentioned periodically, practicing the skill in a varied way improves skill transfer. For instance, if the student struggles with the connection between pressing the foot and the response in the pelvis, you could ask the student to take the feet wider, or turn the toes out, or turn the toes in. Do a few, move on to something else, and the next time the student comes back to it, ask them to try it the original way and see if it's any easier. Repetition with variability

carves out a direct path toward making the skill feel more efficient. It's kind of like trying on different pairs of shoes. If you only try on one pair, how do you know if it's actually comfortable when compared to a different shoe? If, on the other hand, you try on four or five pairs of shoes, there will be a clear standout in the comfort department. You will "know" which pair of shoes feels best based on comparisons to the other shoes. (I recognize this analogy doesn't work if, like me, you spend large amounts of time barefoot or in shoes with minimal support, but you get the idea.)

One of the goals of the nervous system during motor tasks is to reduce motor noise. Motor noise is what happens when a practiced movement appears uncoordinated or is performed in an inefficient way. When a skilled baseball player throws the ball and it veers off course, seemingly out of nowhere, or when you step oddly, losing your balance, those are examples of motor noise (Nguyen & Dingwell 2012). (Motor noise happens in new movements, too. New movements are extra noisy as the neuromuscular system figures out how to do the task with the least amount of effort.)

Motor noise is the result of internal neuromuscular signals and external sources. Research suggests that one way to minimize noise may be to assert control over the proximal joint in a movement task. If, for instance, an individual is struggling with balance tasks, cueing control and stability at the pelvis may reduce performance variability and improve balance more than cueing control and stability at the foot. Both are important, but if you are trying to elicit an immediate change in an individual who would benefit from cueing in both areas, emphasizing proprioception, motor control, and muscular force in the pelvic muscles may give you a more immediate bang for your buck than starting with the feet.

Exercise
Pelvic tilting in tall kneeling

Come into a tall kneeling position, as though you were standing on the knees. If this position is uncomfortable for you, place blankets under the knees, bolstering them up, and think about the points of contact against the floor as being under the kneecap, not directly on the knees (Figure 9.4).

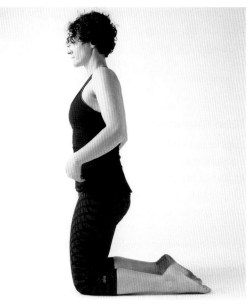

Figure 9.4

Place your fingers on the ASIS. Move the ASIS toward the ribs, and then move them away from your ribs. Do this three or four times, feeling the pelvis move anteriorly and posteriorly (Figures 9.5 and 9.6).

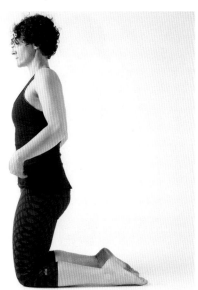

Figure 9.5

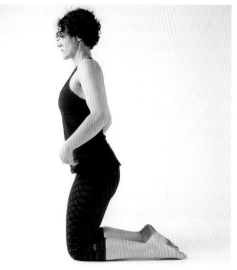

Figure 9.6

Now, rest your hands at your sides. Imagine you have a tail. Move the tail between your legs, and then move the tail away from your legs. Do this three or four times. Feel that action of the pelvis now.

Things to consider and observe

- Which version was easier to perform, initiating the action by moving the bones, or moving an imaginary tail?

- Which direction was easier, moving the pelvis forward or moving the pelvis back?

- Was there a noticeable change in muscular tension when the pelvis shifted posteriorly or anteriorly?

The tall kneeling position is valuable for many reasons. It's an intermediate step for transitioning off the floor and it provides an opportunity to isolate the upper legs. Removing the lower legs and feet often makes it easier to focus on what's happening at the pelvis, just like lowering down to the forearms in a quadruped position can make it easier to feel what happens at the shoulder.

Pelvic tilts performed in a tall kneeling position create awareness around pelvis position and its effect on the muscles in the anterior compartment of the thigh.

When students accomplish pelvis control and mobility in this position, it makes it easier for them to feel where the pelvis is located during more complex positions, such as half kneeling or standing lunge.

Imagery

Imagining a tail is an example of using imagery as an external cue. Mental imagery, which is what happens when you imagine you have a tail, is a psychological activity evoking the physical characteristics of an absent object. It utilizes the senses to create an image in the mind of something specific; in this case, it is the alteration of body schema by adding a tail. The imaginary tail focuses attention on the internal representation of self and takes the focus off of the actual body and how it's moving (Burianova et al. 2013; Krasnow et al. 1997).

There are different forms of imagery that can be used during cueing. Visual imagery refers to imagery that's a memory of a concrete, visually represented item in a student's memory. Kinesthetic imagery is a memory of a kinesthetic event. Both visual and kinesthetic imagery can be used when you ask students to "remember what it looked like when," or "remember what it felt like when."

We have already discussed motor imagery, which is also called direct imagery. It is a nonverbal representation of a movement and occurs when the student imagines performing a specific skill.

Indirect imagery, or metaphorical imagery, is the representation of the desired movement performed with a figure or likeness. It is a form of imagery often used in dance and somatic modalities and is the type of imagery used in the tail example. Though little research has been done on the effectiveness of this type of cueing and teaching, researchers have suggested that more experienced dancers use imagery more frequently and that imagery may enhance dance performance. Whether the use of imagery in a more general movement setting is useful likely depends on the task, the type of imagery, and how receptive the student is to visualization (Nordin & Cumming 2007; Giron et al. 2012).

Using imagery alters how the student executes a specific skill. Imagery can result in more or less tension while performing a movement, depending on how the imagery is cued. Usually, an imaginary tail reduces bracing while performing pelvic tilts. If I wanted to increase the sensation of work, I could ask the student to imagine someone is pushing down on the tail while they move the tail up toward the ceiling.

Lateral movement

During the gait cycle, not only does the pelvis tilt anteriorly and posteriorly, it laterally hikes up, toward the ribs, and down, away from the ribs. These movements happen reciprocally and in the frontal plane, so as one side goes down, the other side goes up, creating the illusion of the pelvis staying level. It's an interesting push/pull that couples with anterior/posterior tilting and rotation to propel you forward.

Exercise
Tall kneeling pelvic elevation and depression

Come into a tall kneeling position. Place your fingers on the ASIS. Reach the right knee into the floor while slightly lifting the left knee off the floor. Switch sides. Go back and forth between the sides three or four times. Feel what's happening beneath the fingers (Figures 9.7 and 9.8).

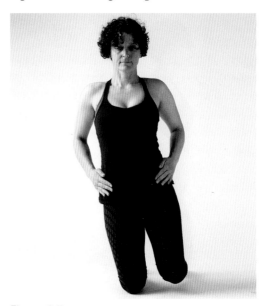

Figure 9.7

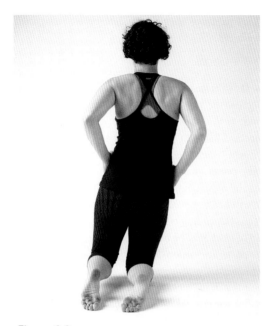

Figure 9.8

Now, imagine you have a tail. Wag your tail slightly to the left and slightly to the right three or four times. Observe how this movement feels and the sensation of the ASIS beneath the fingers.

Things to consider and observe

- Was there clear coordination between the pelvis and knee when the knee reached into the floor? In which direction did the pelvis move?

- Was it easier or more challenging for the student to understand the movement of the pelvis in the knee-reaching position or the tail-wagging position?

The knee-reaching condition is more complex because there is also a balance shift. Any time balance shifts over one side, there is a subtle shift of the center of mass; in individuals who lack strength, the shift becomes less subtle and can resemble more of a lateral lean, kind of like a building that's leaning to one side, as they struggle not to fall over. The wagging-tail condition removes the balance challenge and allows students to focus on just the

subtle change in pelvis position. Because the knee-reach condition integrates balance, it is an excellent warm-up for single-leg balance work, while the tail-wag condition is an excellent warm-up for a pelvis-based movement experience.

The feet and the pelvis

When the feet are in contact with the floor, how they interact with the floor heavily influences what's happening above them, all of the way up into the pelvis (Betsch et al. 2011). The reverse is also true, meaning the position of the pelvis affects what's happening in the feet.

In Chapter 5, I discussed the triangle of the foot. In case you have forgotten, the triangle of the foot refers to the lines connecting the center of the heel to the big toe ball of the foot and the pinkie toe ball of the foot. When the foot is in this position it creates a stable base. During gait, the foot moves away from this position to respond to load and generate force.

One way to illustrate how the foot and pelvis influence each other is to generate different lines of force while the foot is maintaining a stable position using the image of the triangle. The foot becomes a fixed point while the pelvis organizes around it, and the triangular foot utilizes the intrinsic muscles of the foot to maintain the arch. Not only is this position an isometric contraction for the intrinsic foot muscles, it creates a constraint during tasks. A constraint can be thought of as a rule prohibiting you from moving a specific way. This limits the options available for performing the task by reducing the degrees of freedom at the joints above the feet.

Exercise
Connecting the triangles of the feet to the pelvis during pushing

Come into a standing position, preferably in bare feet, with your hands resting comfortably by your sides. Feel the triangles of your feet connecting with the floor.

Bend your knees to about 45° and come into a half squat. Maintaining your triangles, push your feet into the floor, allowing your knees to straighten. Hold that for a couple of seconds and relax. Do this three times.

Come into the same starting position, push your feet into the floor, but don't allow your knees to straighten. Hold for a count of three and relax. Do this three times (Figure 9.9).

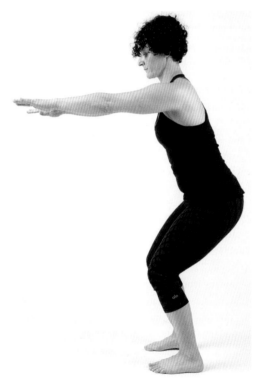

Figure 9.9

Things to consider and observe

- Is the movement of pushing the feet into the floor coordinated with the straightening of the knees?

- Is the student able to maintain the triangle position of the feet or do they change position as the knees straighten? (You will be able to see this if the knees rotate internally or externally during the movement.)

- What happens when the student resists straightening the knee?

- Do the toes stay quiet?

As the feet reach into the floor causing the legs to straighten, the head and torso move up, away from the ground, as the hips extend. There will be a sensation of connection between the feet and the pelvis during the movement (when the feet press, the pelvis shifts position and the center of mass shifts position). When the pelvis resists the movement of the feet pressing into the ground, there will be the sensation of work in the muscles around the hips. Depending on the position of the shins, the sensation of work may be in the anterior portion of the thigh or the posterior portion. Neither is right or wrong, but it is easier to feel the pushing action when the shins are forward of the ankle. If the toes are active during the pushing movement, ask the student if they can perform the same action keeping the toes quiet. Active toes aren't necessarily good or bad, but it's always worthwhile to see if the opposite of the student's habit is available during movements where a low-threshold strategy can be used, such as this one.

If the knees rotate in or out during the movement dynamic part of the movement, observing the feet, particularly the back of the heels, as the student presses the feet into the floor can tell you whether the student struggles to maintain the isometric work at the feet. If the heels collapse in or out, you know the student has neither the strength nor motor control to maintain the foot position during the movement (or maybe both).

Exercise
Connecting the triangles of the feet to pulling

Come into a standing position, preferably in bare feet, with your hands resting comfortably on your hips. Feel the triangles of the feet pressing into the floor.

Shift the hips back so they are behind the feet. The torso will angle forward, and the hands will reach forward (Figure 9.10).

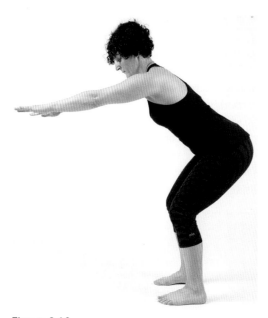

Figure 9.10

Maintaining the sense of the triangle in the feet, reach the feet into the floor and pull the feet toward the wall behind you. The pelvis will shift forward, pulling you back to a standing position.

Try it three or four times, observing the sensation of the feet and the effect the pulling action has on the pelvis.

Things to consider and observe

- Does the forefoot stay on the ground during the movement or does the student lose contact with the forefoot against the ground when the hips shift back?

- Do the two sides of the pelvis move forward at the same rate, or does one side move faster than the other? (This is best observed from the back.)

- Does the movement look connected and integrated, or is it choppy?

Understanding the pulling action of the foot gives the student an opportunity to feel the action of the posterior thigh muscles and how they move the pelvis in a closed-chain position. The ability to both push the feet into the floor and pull them back creates a stable platform to move around (just remember to make sure the feet can leave the floor in a dynamic fashion as well; grounding is wonderful and improves neuroception, but building the strength and balance to feel confident leaving the ground is critical, especially as we age).

Exercise
Connecting the feet with the pelvis in wide-legged stance

Come into a standing position with the feet about one leg's distance apart, so they are wide. Allow the toes to turn out a comfortable amount. (Most people find about 45° feels good, but play with it and see what works best for you.) Allow the knees to angle the same direction as the toes and place your hands in a comfortable position. Maintain the sense of the triangle in the feet (Figure 9.11).

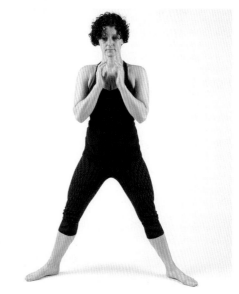

Figure 9.11

Pull the heels toward each other. Allow the knees to bend as the heels pull toward each other. Reach the heels into the floor and away from each other. Allow the knees to straighten. Do this three or four times, holding the hips lowered position for three or four breaths on the last one. Feel the feet interacting with the floor and see if you can find the place between the transition of pulling and reaching to feel maximally supported (Figure 9.12).

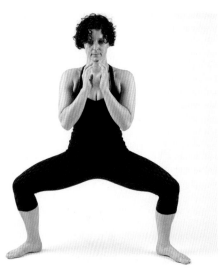

Figure 9.12

Things to consider and observe

- Was there coordination between pulling the heels toward each other, the knees bending, and the pelvis moving down?

- Did the knees stay oriented in the same angle as the toes?

- Was there a sensation of work in the pelvic floor or the muscles in the legs?

The externally rotated feet and femur position subtly changes the position of the pelvis, externally rotating each hemipelvis. Cueing breath in this position can improve the student's relationship between breathing and the pelvic floor (the inhale will create a sense of fullness in the pelvic floor, while the exhale will create the sensation of the pelvic floor moving up and contracting). Cueing the movement from the feet allows the lower extremity to self-organize without the student overthinking the movement, which can be beneficial for exposing the student to a (possibly) new position.

Exercise
Using the feet to shift the pelvis

Come into a standing position with the feet slightly wider than one leg's distance apart. Allow the toes to turn out a comfortable amount. Place the hands in a comfortable position and maintain the sense of the triangle in the feet (Figure 9.13).

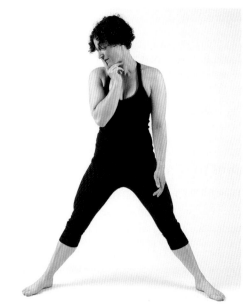

Figure 9.13

Pull the inside of the right foot toward the left foot. Allow the right knee to bend and the pelvis to shift to the right (Figures 9.14 and 9.15).

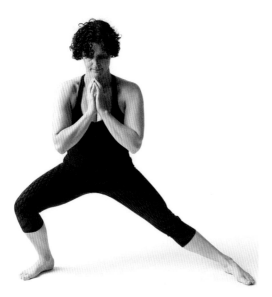

Figure 9.14

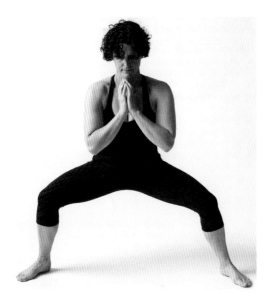

Figure 9.15

Pull the inside of the left foot toward the right foot, allowing the left knee to bend and the pelvis to shift to the left (Figure 9.16).

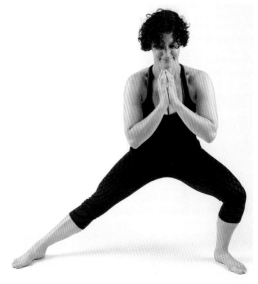

Figure 9.16

Go back and forth between the two positions four or five times, feeling how the feet determine which direction the pelvis shifts.

Things to consider and observe

- Is the student able to maintain the connection between the triangle of the feet and the pelvis throughout the movement?

- Is one side more fluid than the other?

- Does the student stay low to shift or does the student lift out of it? (Neither is right or wrong. It's just interesting to observe which strategy is used.)

Using the feet to direct the shifting of the pelvis in this position usually creates natural stability in the torso. However, if the student is struggling with torso stability, ask the student to hold a yoga block or weight with the hands in the center of the chest. This acts as a constraint and naturally prevents excessive movement in the torso. The more secure the student is in their feet, the more efficient the movement will look.

The last two exercises favored an externally rotated hemipelvis. What if the student already understands how to perform this action? Then, it may be beneficial to teach the student how to internally rotate the pelvis. An easy way to do this is explored in the next exercise.

Exercise
Closing the ASIS and the effect on the feet

Come into a comfortable standing position. Observe the sensation of your pelvis. Is it forward of your heels? Or back behind your heels? Or maybe it's somewhere in between? Move it forward and back a few times until you feel like it's in a "neutral" position.

Feel the sensation of your feet against the ground, observing how they connect with the floor.

Place your fingers on your ASIS. Imagine there is a string between your fingers that is lightly being pulled taut, as though the distance between your two hands was shortening. Relax.

Perform this action three or four times. Observe what happens in the feet as you do this. Does the way they are connecting to the ground change?

Things to consider and observe

- Was the student able to feel a subtle shift beneath their fingers or in their feet?

- Did the student feel the sensation of work in the abdominals or legs?

- Was the student able to keep the rest of the body quiet and breathe as they performed the action?

The action of the two ASIS lightly pulling toward each other internally rotates the pelvis, which means it internally rotates the femurs and internally rotates the tibia. If this is opposite a student's habit, the first time they perform the action is often accompanied by the sensation of work in the abdominals and/or legs. Using the metaphorical image of the string generally causes the student to perform the movement in a softer way, which is the goal of this particular movement. Though it's subtle, as you will see in the case study below, it can have a profound effect on a person's experience of movement in the pelvis and lower extremity. It also brings awareness of the location of the pelvis in space, which is useful when teaching movements like a split stance or lunge position where the goal is a square or closed pelvis/hip orientation.

Case study

A client fell and injured the medial collateral ligament in her knee. The orthopedic surgeon encouraged her to let it heal rather than do surgery.

With time, it healed, but it would still give her twinges occasionally when she went for her daily four-mile walk. I suggested she try thinking about bringing the ASIS together when she walked to see if that helped. This particular client had a strong habit of externally rotating both the two sides of the pelvis and the lower extremities. I wondered if bringing awareness to the opposite position would make a difference.

She came in the following week, beaming. "The pain is gone! Bringing the two bony points on the front of the pelvis together fixed it. Thank you!"

She still uses the cue to this day, years later, if she feels discomfort in her knee. Changing what happens at one area alters movement throughout the musculoskeletal system, creating a different movement pattern and, it is hoped, a new experience.

During the majority of the gait cycle, one leg is forward while one leg is back. The position of the hemipelvis depends on which part of the gait cycle the leg is in. About 80% of the time, the pelvis is in an anterior pelvic tilt. It's in a posterior pelvic tilt directly following initial contact with the stance leg (the stance leg refers to the foot that is in contact with the ground). Following contact, the stance phase hemipelvis drops while the swing phase hemipelvis hikes. For example, as the right foot makes initial contact with the ground, the right ASIS is forward of the left ASIS, the right hemipelvis is rotating forward, and the left hemipelvis rotates backward. The right hemipelvis moves down toward the ground as the pelvis shifts over the right leg; as the right leg prepares to leave the ground, the right hemipelvis begins to elevate and rotate forward.

This point during the walking gait where both legs are on the ground and the right foot prepares to leave the ground, shifting the right hemipelvis to a forward rotation and the left hemipelvis to a backward rotation is reliant on adequate strength and mobility in both sides of the pelvis and both legs. Fortunately, this position resembles the split stance or lunge position and can be explored a number of ways to help students feel the relationships between the two sides of the pelvis and the feet (Lewis et al. 2017).

Exercise
Split stance pelvic rotation

Come into a standing position with the legs split so the left leg is forward with the knee bent and the right leg is back and straight, as though you had just taken a large step. Keep both heels on the floor. Place your fingers on the ASIS.

Let the right hemipelvis rotate back and forward a few times. The area under your fingers will move back and forth alternately. As you do this, the left hemipelvis rotates in the opposite direction. Observe how that feels in the legs (Figure 9.17).

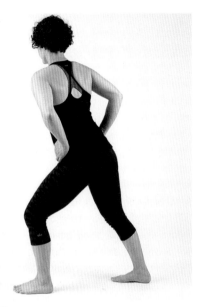

Figure 9.17

Now, lift the right heel off the ground, but keep everything else the same. Perform the same movement, letting the right hemipelvis rotate back and forward. Do this a few times, shake out your legs, and then switch sides (Figure 9.18).

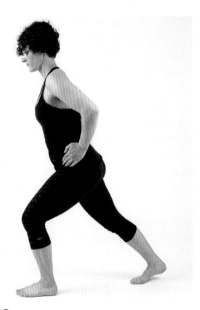

Figure 9.18

Things to consider and observe

- Is it easier for the student to rotate the pelvis with the heel up or down?

- Was one side easier than the other?

- Was the torso completely vertical or did it angle forward?

- Was the student able to maintain a flexed knee or did it extend as the pelvis rotated?

Most people find it easier to rotate the pelvis with the back heel lifted. When the back heel is on the floor, it acts as a constraint, limiting the degrees of freedom.

If the student maintains a vertical torso or extends the front knee as they rotate, the student is avoiding placing load in the front leg. This may be a habit that developed to avoid the sensation of work, it may be a motor control issue, or if there has ever been an injury or surgery, it may be habit that developed to avoid discomfort. Assuming there is no longer any discomfort present, cueing the student to actively push the front foot into the ground and allow the torso to come forward so they can feel the sensation of work in the stance leg helps the student develop a stronger connection with the leg while it is supporting the majority of the body's weight.

Split stance positions are a great way to introduce movements that resemble different phases of gait; they are also an effective way to work on closed-chain hip mobility. Whenever the pelvis is rotating around a fixed foot, it's rotating over the head of the femur, facilitating movement in the joint. To work on open-chain hip mobility, the pelvis remains fixed and the thigh moves around the pelvis.

Exercise
Supine open-chain hip mobility

Lie on your back with the knees bent and the feet flat on the floor. Place your fingers on your ASIS. Without allowing the ASIS to move, ground the left foot and reach the right leg out so it's straight and resting on the ground.

Turn the right knee to the right and bend it, sliding the right knee up, still not allowing the ASIS to move beneath the fingers. Straighten the right knee and rotate the knee toward the ceiling. Play with this three or four times (Figure 9.19).

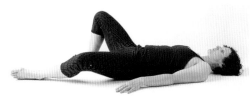

Figure 9.19

Now, still grounding the left foot and not allowing the ASIS to move, pick the right foot off the floor so the knee is bent and over the right hip. Move the right knee in different directions. You can move it away from the midline of the body, bring it toward the midline of the body, rotate it out, rotate it in, move it away from the body so the leg straightens, bring it toward the body so the knee bends more, and make circles with remain still beneath the fingertips. Spend about 45–60 seconds exploring different ways to move the knee.

Once you have finished, set the right foot down. Spend a moment observing the sensation in the hips (Figure 9.20).

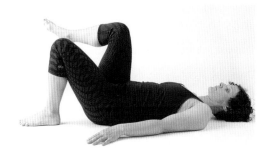

Figure 9.20

Things to consider and observe

- Was the student able to keep the pelvis still while they moved the leg?

- Was it easier for the student to keep the pelvis still while the leg was extended and on the floor or while the foot was off the ground?

- Which positions appeared easier and more coordinated, or was there fluidity throughout the movement?

If the student struggles to keep the pelvis still while moving the leg, the student may not understand what it feels like to keep the pelvis still or how to keep the pelvis still, making it a motor control issue. The student may also not have the strength to keep the pelvis still while moving the leg, which would make it a stability issue. The student may also have a specific reason (for example, hip pain) that limits the amount of accessible movement at the hip. Asking the student what they are experiencing, either as they perform the movement or after they have finished, can help you determine the best course of action. Assuming there is no pain or discomfort in the hip joint or pelvis while performing the movements, basic stability drills that require a fixed pelvis, like a forearm plank or supine core stability drills, can give the student the proprioceptive information needed to make a correction and differentiate movement between the pelvis and the hip.

Researchers speculate that there may be a connection between hip function and low back pain, specifically that lack of sufficient hip mobility may contribute to low back pain. The exact mechanisms behind why this would occur remain unclear but imagine for a moment that every time you moved your left leg, no matter how big or small the motion, the left hemipelvis moved as well. Not only is that a lot of extra work, it also means force is being distributed in a less efficient way. Taking the time to help students feel and understand the difference between the hip and the pelvis allows the entire neuromuscular system to work more efficiently and makes the pelvis and torso area feel more stable (Harris-Hayes et al. 2009). Remember that one way to improve proprioception is through force; it requires muscular force to prevent pelvic movement during open-chain hip movement, improving proprioception.

I mentioned earlier that during the stance phase of the gait cycle, the foot presses down and the hip drops, while the swing leg hip hikes. What happens if the hip hikes on the stance leg during the initial stance phase of gait? What does that mean?

Often, this comes from the inability of the foot to generate force down as it connects with the ground. Think back to the exercise we did earlier where the knees were bent, the feet pressed down, the knees straightened, and the torso moved up. If the knees were to remain bent (which you also tried), there would be a sense of work in the muscles in the leg and pelvis.

Initial stance functions in a similar way. Pretend the left leg is in the early stages of stance and the left foot is pressing into the ground. The pressing of the foot happens first, causing a cascade of events, including the left hemipelvis subtly dropping and the torso moving up, away from the pelvis. There is a response throughout the spine, including thoracic spine rotation to the left as the left arm swings back and the right arm swings forward. Walking and running are very dynamic, coordinated movements requiring both stability and mobility.

If the left foot is unable to actively press into the floor, the neuromuscular system will coordinate in a less efficient manner. In this example, without the left foot driving force down, the left hemipelvis has nothing to prevent it from swinging out to the side as momentum from the pelvis is used to move over the stance leg.

This can be highlighted more clearly when you place the legs in a split stance position with the front foot elevated on a small step. As the front foot presses into the step, this causes the same chain of events that happens during gait, including the front hemipelvis moving the same direction of the foot (down) as the head moves up toward the ceiling.

Exercise

Split stance with step to highlight pelvic movement

If you have a shallow step, face the step, and place the right foot on the step. If you don't have a step, a book or yoga block will do.

Place your fingers on the ASIS and square the hips. Keeping the right knee bent, press the right foot down, transferring weight to the right foot as the left heel begins to lift off the ground. Observe what happens to the pelvis underneath the right fingers. Hold for a count of three and then relax. Perform this movement three or four times and switch sides (Figure 9.21).

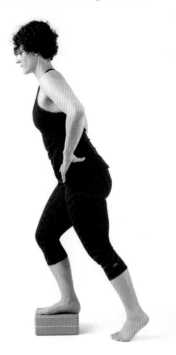

Figure 9.21

Things to consider and observe

- Can you feel the front foot pressing down?
- Does the front hemipelvis hike up or does it move down?
- Does the back hemipelvis begin to move forward and up when the heel lifts off the ground?
- Is there a sensation of work anywhere?

If the student is able to generate force downward with the front foot, the pelvis will appear visually even. The subtle actions occurring as the front hemipelvis drops and the back hemipelvis begins to hike gives the illusion of symmetry, though, as we know, nothing is ever truly symmetrical. If the student is unable to generate downward force with the front foot in this position, the pelvis will appear uneven. The inability to generate force will make movements like single-leg squat variations and stepping variations challenging. While I am emphasizing the foot, the muscles of the abdominals are responsible for balancing the movement above the pelvis, so, really, total body integration is required for single-leg, bent-knee skills to occur in a coordinated fashion. This exercise can be a great neuromuscular warm-up for single-leg squat drills or for asymmetrical squatting drills. If you press down throughout the range of motion and emphasize the connection between the stance leg (or both feet, if it's a symmetrical squat pattern) it improves neuroception. (It was previously established that it feels safer to perform a movement when there is a firm base of support connecting with the ground.) This cue may also improve balance, coordination, and kinesthetic awareness, due to the emphasis on force, which requires muscular effort.

A friend of mine who was sexually assaulted several years ago once described the lower abdominal area between the ASIS in front of the pelvis as a black hole, devoid of feeling. I have witnessed similar disconnections in others over the years, and while I don't always know why the student is disembodied, dissociation from the pelvis visibly impacts the student's movement. The ability to control the pelvis influences the center of mass and, as you have learned, is critical for efficient transfer of force from the lower limb to the torso. Learning to move gently and softly in the pelvis is just as important as learning to generate force and power. When someone lacks the kinesthetic awareness of the pelvis or hasn't incorporated it fully into their body schema, movement throughout the entire body will be affected.

The goal of the movement practitioner, then, is to invite movement that is pain free and gentle at first, giving the student the opportunity to establish connections. Maybe the pelvis is cued; maybe it isn't. Interoceptive cues have a place, but if you know the student experienced trauma in the past, taking the focus outside the self can be a way to explore movement in a way that may feel safer; as discussed in Chapter 4, a safe environment leads to more fluid, easeful movement. This doesn't mean things that are challenging should be avoided; it does, however, suggest spending a few minutes to improve the individual's kinesthetic awareness of the pelvis and how it interacts with the rest of the body may set the individual up for success in more complex, challenging movements later. Strength is predicated on stability, motor control, and mobility; these three pieces can be developed individually or together, depending on the student's interests and needs.

Connections are meant to be explored. Using the basic concepts of the sense of physical self and its relation with the world begins to chip away at the belief that the mind and body are separate and re-establish integration. Connections can be explored in endless ways; the exercises illustrated in this chapter and throughout the book are just examples. As long as you, the teacher, have a clear idea of the student's goals for a movement practice, the possibilities for teaching the concepts are limited only by your imagination.

References

Betsch M, Schneppendahl J, Dor L, Jungbluth P, Grassman JP, Windolf J, Thelen S, Hakimi M, Rapp W, and Wild M (2011) Influence of foot positions on the spine and pelvis. Arthritis Care Research 63 (12) 1,758–1,765.

Booth J and Morris J (2019) The sacroiliac – victim or culprit. Best Practice & Research Clinical Rheumatology 33 88–101.

Breit S, Kupferberg A, Rogler G, and Hasler G (2018) Vagus nerve as modulator of the brain–gut axis in psychiatric and inflammatory disorders. Frontiers in Psychiatry 9 (44) 1–15.

Burianova H, Marstaller L, Sowman P, Tesan G, Rich AN, Williams M, Savage G, and Johnson BW (2013) Multimodal functional imaging of motor imagery using a novel paradigm. Neuroimage 71 50–58.

Chan CW and Rudins A (1994) Foot biomechanics during walking and running. Mayo Clinic Proceedings 69 (5) 448–461.

Giron EC, McIsaac T, and Nilsen D (2012) Effects of kinesthetic versus visual imagery practice on two technical dance movements: A pilot study. Journal of Dance and Medical Science 16 (1) 35–38.

Gold M and Varacallo M (2019) Anatomy, bony pelvis and lower limb: Hip joint. Treasure Island, FL: StatPcarls.

Hagan CE, Bolon B, and Keene CD (2012) Nervous system, in Treuting PM, Dintzis, SM, and Montine KS (eds) Comparative anatomy and histology: A mouse and human atlas. London, UK: Academic Press.

Harris-Hayes M, Sahrmann SA, and Van Dillen LR (2009) Relationship between the hip and low back pain in athletes who participate in rotation-related sports. Journal of Sport Rehabilitation 18 (1) 60–75.

Juunger MJ, ter Meulen BC, Weinstein HC, and Ostelo RWJG. (2019) Inflammatory biomarkers in patients with sciatica: A systematic review. BMC Musculoskeletal Disorders 20 (156) 1–9.

Krasnow DH, Chatfield SJ, Barr S, Jensen JL, and Dufek JS (1997) Imagery and conditioning practices for dancers. Dance Research Journal 29 (1) 16–20.

Lewis CL, Laudicina NM, Khuu A, and Loverro KI (2017) The human pelvis: Variation in structure and function during gait. The Anatomical Record 300 633–642.

Musielak B, Jozwiak M, Rychlik M, Chen BP-J, Idzior M, and Grzegorzewski A (2016) Does hemipelvis structure and position influence acetabulum orientation? BMC Musculoskeletal Disorders 17 (131) 1–7.

Nguyen HP and Dingwell JB (2012) Proximal versus distal control of two-joint planar reaching movements in the presence of neuromuscular noise. Journal of Biomechanical Engineering 134 (6), 061007.

Nordin SM and Cumming J (2007) Where, when, and how: A quantitative account of dance imagery. Research Quarterly for Exercise & Sport 78 (4) 390–395.

Park H and Han D (2015) The effect of the correlation between the contraction of the pelvic floor muscles and diaphragmatic motion during breathing. Journal of Physical Therapy Science 27 (7) 2,113–2,115.

Rad LS, Babolhavaeji F, and Babolhavaeji E (2012) A comparison of blocked and random practice on acquisition of swimming skills. European Journal of Experimental Biology 2 (6) 2,073–2,076.

Speer LM, Mushkbar S, and Erbele T (2016) Chronic pelvic pain in women. American Family Physician 93 (5) 380–387.

Udoji MA and Ness TJ (2013) New directions in the treatment of pelvic pain. Pain Management 3 (5) 387–394.

Vleeming A, Schuenke MD, Masi AT, Carreiro JE, Danneels L, and Williard FH (2012) The sacroiliac joint: An overview of its anatomy, function and potential clinical implications. Journal of Anatomy 221 537–567.

Conclusion

We each have our own movement fingerprint that expresses who we are to the world. This uniqueness creates an individualized way of embodying playfulness, emotion, and autonomy. Reminding people that there is no right or wrong way to move opens a door for more movement freedom. Inspiring curiosity in the connections between different areas of the body and viewing movement and the physical awareness of the body as skills that can be cultivated with practice taps into something more meaningful than endless sets and reps, static positions, or specific, choreographed movement. While those pieces help develop physical stamina and strength, they don't necessarily create a deeper connection between the student and their body, two entities that aren't separate. Developing a sense of embodiment gives people access to feeling more secure and stable in their daily lives.

One of the things I find interesting in working with people is that as they begin to realize the connections explored on these pages, the more curious they become about what their bodies are capable of doing. Movement creates more movement, even if the movement is subtle at first. There is no shortage of information regarding the importance of physical activity, but the reality is people hurt, they don't have energy, or they don't want to prioritize it because there is a shortage of time in everyone's days. Making small steps toward establishing a mind–body connection can make a huge difference in a person's quality of life and their ability to interact with the world, and one another, in a meaningful way.

Spend time asking questions and listening, offering opportunities for self-reflection. The long-term effects of learning may come when you least expect it. Awareness, after all, is the first step to change.

Appendices

Appendix 1 Low back pain

When you begin working with someone who experiences chronic low back pain and has been cleared by a medical professional to begin a movement program, keep the following points in mind:

Listen to the student. Ask what positions are uncomfortable and when they notice the pain most. If the positions are ones that are necessary for activities of daily living, like standing or sitting, play with different positions until you find one that is comfortable. If there is a specific movement that is provoking, like bending over, spend time developing strength and awareness in positions that resemble bending over, but aren't actually bending over. Examples are supine straight leg flexion, seated straight leg flexion, and standing hip flexion with the torso hinged forward a small amount. You can move in and out of these positions actively; you can cue them to be easeful or strong; and you can incorporate isometrics in various places to improve strength and proprioception, and reduce the sensation of threat. Gradually, incorporate movements such as bending forward to touch a high box or chair. If it doesn't provoke pain, play with touching the box in different positions, gradually making the box lower as confidence increases.

Pay attention to the center of mass. If the student moves away from the center of mass (COM), develop a connection using strength and stability exercises (external load tends to work well for this). Cue the center of mass frequently, so the student begins to understand where the COM is located and how that area provides support. Two areas that can help maintain connection to COM are the ribs and the pelvis.

If there is fear or a disconnection with the pelvis, start with small movements after trust has been established (so maybe not in the first or even the fifth session). Perhaps use visualization before cueing pelvis-specific movement. Remember, interoceptive/internal cues may not initially be the best choice with individuals who have fear or anxiety around movement in a specific area. Think creatively and find ways to use external cues to create kinesthetic awareness and improve strength.

If someone keeps the spine rigid during movement, find ways to increase mobility.

If someone has a significant amount of postural sway and the spine moves a lot during movement, find ways to increase strength.

Use the concept of graded exposure to improve tolerance and don't be afraid to start with introducing specific movements on a small scale, giving the student time to assimilate new ways of using the body. Fatigue alters movement patterns; for deconditioned individuals, fatigue sets in sooner than you may expect. Both less is more and quality versus quantity should be applied, and, remember, if the student has done nothing for the last four years, performing an exercise or skill four times is more than they did yesterday. Strength, coordination, and mobility improve with time. There is no rush, and as a student's confidence increases, so, too, will their ability to approach more challenging positions.

Be aware of the language you use. Words like "dysfunction," "imbalance," "tightness," and "weakness" all imply there is something wrong with the student's physicality and their ability to learn. Use words that cultivate a growth mindset when you teach, reminding students they are capable and strong.

Appendices

Appendix 2 Hypermobility

Training students with benign joint hypermobility, or symptomatic joint hypermobility, requires listening, paying attention, and focusing the student's attention. Remember that hypermobility is correlated with lack of confidence in balance, anxiety, and heightened interoception; movement interventions should emphasize strength, focused attention on tasks or activities rather than internal senses, and a growth mindset. Things to keep in mind while working with these students include:

How does the student use their feet? Are they providing stability or does the student struggle to generate downward force with the feet?

Can the student isolate movement at specific joints or does the student achieve movement by shifting in the torso, pelvis, or elsewhere?

Are you using externally based tasks and cues to accomplish the desired effect? How is the student responding to the cues?

Can the student feel the sensation of work in various positions? Remember, force improves proprioception. For these individuals, feeling the sensation of work and how the muscles support the joints is important, so while cueing may be primarily externally based, drawing attention to the internal experience can support awareness.

Is the student sensitive to sensation that is being interpreted as pain? If so, start with a low rep/set schema and build up from there.

How does a constraint, such as an external load, change the student's movement strategy?

Goals for the hypermobile student

- Increase strength.

- Increase kinesthetic awareness.

- Increase balance.

Reduce fear around movement by using thoughtful regressions and paying attention to position. (These individuals have a plethora of movement options available. Teaching these individuals how to isolate movement and how to recover from perturbations is critical for long-term success.)

Appendices

Appendix 3 Assessment checklist

Assessing can (and should) be done in a relaxed manner so the student doesn't feel judged. Observing movements while a student moves in a natural way can reveal more about the student's habits than a specified assessment. Some things to notice: how does the student stand while chatting with you? Is one hip oriented back of the other? Do the knees lock? Does the pelvis thrust forward or back?

In what direction is the head oriented when the student walks in to your studio? (Does the student look down while walking, out toward the horizon, or up toward the sky?)

What is the natural orientation of the feet when the student is supine, with the knees bent and the feet flat? Do the toes angle in? Out? Is one foot forward of the other?

When the student stands on one leg, does the inside of the stabilizing foot move toward the floor or away from the floor?

When the student squats, what does it look like from the back? Does one hip move more rapidly up or down than the other? Does the pelvis shift in the frontal plane? Or rotate in the transverse plane? Or does part of the foot move away from the ground? Or toward the ground?

When the student raises an arm in the sagittal plane, is there a shift in the torso? What about when the student raises an arm in the frontal plane?

When the student reaches an arm forward, does the pelvis shift?

Can the student place weight in the center of the heel and keep it there while squatting (either double or single leg; it's good to observe both)?

What does the spine do when the forearms or hands are loaded against a wall? (Think prone plank position at the wall.) What happens when one arm moves and the student stabilizes on one hand in this position? How does the spine respond?

Assessments are simply observations. These are some of the things I look at while watching someone move. The interventions I use depend on what I observe and what the student tells me with regards to discomfort or perceived stiffness or weakness. Because formal assessments can be perceived as judgment, I prefer to introduce movements and observe. Any movement can be used as an opportunity for observation to learn more about the movement strategies of the person in front of you.

INDEX